CONTEMPORARY MANAGEMENT IN INTERNAL MEDICINE

JAY H. STEIN, MD, Editor-in-Chief

Professor and Chairman
The Dan F. Parman Distinguished Chair in Medicine
Department of Medicine
The University of Texas
Health Science Center at San Antonio
San Antonio, Texas

EDITORIAL BOARD

CHURCHILL LIVINGSTONE
New York, Edinburgh, London, Melbourne, Tokyo 1991

FORTHCOMING ISSUES

GRANULOMATOUS INFECTIONS

DWIGHT M. WILLIAMS, MD
Editor

Professor
Department of Medicine
Division of Infectious Diseases
University of Texas
Health Science Center at San Antonio
Associate Chief of Education
Audie L. Murphy Memorial Veterans Hospital
San Antonio, Texas

CHURCHILL LIVINGSTONE
New York, Edinburgh, London, Melbourne, Tokyo 1991

ISSN: 1050-9607
ISBN 0-443-08837-3

Direct subscription orders, changes of address, and claims for missing issues (within five months of publication) to Churchill Livingstone Inc. (650 Avenue of the Americas, New York, NY 10011). In Japan, contact Nankodo Co., Ltd., 42-6, Hongo 3-chome, Bunkyo-ku, Tokyo 113, Japan.

The authors, editors, and publisher have exerted every effort to ensure that drug selection and dosage and descriptions of instruments and recommendations for their use set forth in all articles appearing in *Contemporary Management in Internal Medicine* are in accord with current recommendations and practice at the time of publication. However, many considerations necessitate caution in applying in practice any information appearing in *Contemporary Management in Internal Medicine*. The reader is advised to check package inserts for each drug for indications and dosages and the descriptions provided by instrument manufacturers for warnings and precautions.

The publishers have made every effort to trace the copyright holders for borrowed material. If they have inadvertently overlooked any, they will be pleased to make the necessary arrangements at the first opportunity.

Printed in the United States of America

Volume 2 Number 1
First published in 1991

CONTRIBUTING AUTHORS

John R. Graybill, MD
Professor
Department of Medicine
Division of Infectious Diseases
University of Texas
Health Science Center at San Antonio
San Antonio, Texas

Neil M. Ampel, MD
Staff Physician
Medical Service
Section of Infectious Disease (111)
Veterans Administration Medical Center
Associate Professor
Department of Medicine
University of Arizona
Health Sciences Center
Tucson, Arizona

Philip C. Johnson, MD
Director, Division of General Internal Medicine
University of Texas
Health Science Center at Houston
Houston, Texas

Patricia Kay Sharkey, MD
Assistant Professor
Department of Medicine
Division of Infectious Diseases
University of Texas
Health Science Center at San Antonio
San Antonio, Texas

Robert A. Zajac, MD
Clinical Assistant Professor
Department of Medicine
University of Texas
Health Science Center at San Antonio
San Antonio, Texas

Gregory P. Melcher, MD
Chief, Infectious Diseases Service
Wilford Hall Medical Center
Lackland AFB
Clinical Associate Professor
Department of Medicine
University of Texas
Health Science Center at San Antonio
San Antonio, Texas

Jean A. Smith, MD
Assistant Professor
Department of Medicine
Division of Infectious Diseases
University of Texas
Health Science Center at San Antonio
San Antonio, Texas

GRANULOMATOUS INFECTIONS

CONTENTS

Volume 2   Number 1

GRANULOMATOUS INFECTIONS

PREFACE

In an era of growing numbers of immunosuppressed patients, granulomatous infections are becoming increasingly important both as primary infections and as reactivation disease. In this issue of *Contemporary Management in Internal Medicine* are six chapters dealing with fungal and mycobacterial granulomatous infections. Dr. J. Richard Graybill has produced an encyclopedic treatise on the subject of treatment of fungal infection in general. Dr. Neil Ampel has dealt with coccidioidomycosis in particular, while Dr. Johnson has provided an in-depth review of histoplasmosis. Frequently, the clinician is confronted with apparent "aseptic" meningitis, which may be due to a granulomatous process. Dr. Sharkey has written an extensive review of the topic, including suggested diagnostic modalities and empiric therapy. Mycobacterial infection is becoming an increasing management problem in an era of AIDS. Drs. Melcher and Zajac have reviewed new information on the diagnosis and treatment of pulmonary tuberculosis, while Dr. Smith has discussed mycobacterial infection (both typical and atypical) in AIDS. New infection control information related to mycobacterial infection is covered in these chapters as well. It is hoped that this issue will provide a useful synthesis of the large amount of new information that has recently become available concerning the pathogenesis, diagnosis, and treatment of granulomatous infections.

I would like to thank each of the authors for his or her contribution, and Connie Stahl, MS, for her excellent technical assistance.

Dwight M. Williams, MD

ANTIFUNGAL THERAPY FOR SYSTEMIC MYCOSES

JOHN R. GRAYBILL, MD

HISTORICAL PERSPECTIVE

For many years the systemic mycotic infections were thought to be few in number and not worthy of attention from the pharmaceutical industry. The major mycoses of the 1960s were divided into the so-called dimorphic endemic mycoses and the opportunists. Of the four dimorphic endemic mycoses, infection with *Histoplasma capsulatum* and *Blastomyces dermatitidis* occurs in the midwestern and southeastern United States, while *Coccidioides immitis* ranges from Texas to California and down through Mexico and, in scattered endemic foci, to Argentina. *Paracoccidioides brasiliensis* ranges from Mexico through Argentina. These infections are not transmitted man to man, and in general the infected human either remained asymptomatic or developed a transient pneumonia that resolved on its own. Only infrequently did these infections take the course of disseminated progressive disease.

In contrast, there was another group of mycoses brought together under the name "opportunists." These were further grouped according to whether they took advantage of defects in cell-mediated immunity or phagocyte function. These fungi are commonly commensal organisms living on the skin or, occasionally, on mucous membranes, in the gastrointestinal tract, or contaminating respiratory secretions. Among the former is *Cryptococcus neoformans*, which (in the United States) caused 300–400 cases of meningitis per year before 1980, and among the latter are *Candida* species, *Aspergillus* species, and the zygomycetes. These infections were associated with defective phagocyte function, neutropenia, and in the case of zygomycetes, the hyperglycemia and acidosis associated with uncontrolled diabetes mellitus.

The above reflected the era of the "Good Old Days," in which mycoses were few and mycologists fewer, and the major interests of mycologists were directed at the much more common but less dangerous dermatomycoses. The advent of amphotericin B in the late 1950s provided one highly effective (albeit highly toxic), broad-spectrum antifungal drug that could be used against most of the systemic mycoses, and a decade later the addition of flucytosine augmented the therapeutic options for candidiasis, cryptococcosis, and possibly aspergillosis and chromoblastomycosis.

Patients who otherwise would have succumbed to primary illness or bacterial infection survived in precarious health, such that fungal "opportunists" had the opportunity to exploit broad gaps in host defense.

In the 1970s the state of torpor was terminated by the development of a broad range of cytotoxic and immunosuppressive drugs, increasingly aggressive use of intensive care units, and an ever-broadening spectrum of antibacterial drugs. Patients who otherwise would have succumbed to primary illness or bacterial infection survived long enough and in precarious enough health such that fungal "opportunists" had the opportunity to exploit broad gaps in host defenses. Candidemia and invasive aspergillosis became "household words," and took an increasingly high toll of immunosuppressed patients. Further, new pathogens such as *Fusarium* and *Trichosporon* entered the arena as opportunists in the leukopenic patient.

Histoplasmosis and coccidioidomycosis are appearing with such frequency in AIDS patients that their designation as primary endemic mycosis is blurring.

The 1980s have been marked by continuing expansion of the above-mentioned practices as well as the AIDS pandemic. The mycologic consequences of this were a marked increase in the numbers of patients with mucosal infections of *Candida* organisms in the form of thrush, esophagitis, and now, perhaps diarrhea. *Candida* organisms caused morbidity frequently and mortality rarely. *C neoformans*, a formerly rare pathogen, now infects as many as 6–12% of Americans with AIDS and may be three times as frequent in African patients with AIDS.[1-3] *H capsulatum*, formerly a rare pathogen of the immunodepressed host, increased in frequency to as much as 5% in endemic areas,[4] while coccidioidomycosis has assumed a frequency of almost 3% in HIV-infected patients residing in Tucson, Arizona, a "capital" of the endemic area. Both histoplasmosis and coccidioidomycosis are appearing with such frequency in AIDS patients that their designation as primary endemic mycosis is blurring; they are becoming increasingly recognized as opportunistic infections in the setting of AIDS. It is curious that despite the almost overlapping of its endemic zone with histoplasmosis, blastomycosis is still very rare in AIDS patients, with only 12 patients reported in the most recent survey.[5]

Ketoconazole revolutionized the world of systemic antifungal therapy.

All of these events increased both the frequency and the severity of the systemic mycoses, and the need for more effective and less toxic therapeutic options rapidly came to the fore. In 1979 Janssen introduced ketoconazole, a broad-spectrum, orally absorbed imidazole antifungal. Ketoconazole was effective for such severe diseases as disseminated histoplasmosis, yet safe enough to use for onychomycosis. Ketoconazole revolutionized the world of systemic antifungal therapy. This chapter will concentrate on the most recent developments of new antifungals, emphasizing our present status and the alternatives that may be available to us in the 1990s.[6] Following a review of the specific classes of antifungals, specific fungal infections will be considered with present recommendations for therapy and how these might change in the future.

CHARACTERIZATION OF ANTIFUNGALS

Polyenes

The polyene antifungals are characterized by long carbon chains linked by divalent "ene" bonds. Amphotericin B has been utilized for 3 decades for a wide variety of infections. Despite its use for many years, we are still learning how amphotericin B exerts its antifungal activity, what the proper dosing regimens are for patients with a variety of mycoses, and how to minimize toxicity.[7]

The mechanism of polyene antifungal drugs derives from the drugs' preferential binding to ergosterol of fungal cell membranes. This causes loss of osmotic integrity and leaking of intracellular constituents, including potassium. Loss of membrane integrity was for some time thought to be the chief mechanism responsible for antifungal activity, but we now know that cidal activity derives from intracellular release of oxygen radicals and intracellular oxidative processes.[7] Amphotericin B binds to proteins and to cholesterol and has been found to cause significant toxicity based on this mechanism. The slow leaching of potassium in renal tubular cells may be due to this process, with resultant hypokalemia. Rapid infusion of amphotericin B in patients with renal failure causes a paradoxical elevation in serum potassium, probably from leakage of erythrocytes or muscle or other cells.[8]

Amphotericin B is poorly soluble in water and is currently available as a colloidal suspension in deoxycholate (Fungizone, Squibb). Amphotericin B is not readily absorbed after oral administration and must be given by local irrigation (50 mg/L water), intravenous infusion (commonly up to 1 mg/kg), or intrathecal injection (commonly 0.5 mg 3 times/wk). The drug rapidly separates from the vehicle after intravenous infusion, and up to 30% is excreted by hepatobiliary and renal routes.[9,10] The fate of the remainder is uncertain. Infusion time of amphotericin B was commonly 4–6 hours a decade ago, but practice has changed to increase the rate of infusion to as little as 1 hour. In a few patients this can be quite dangerous, resulting in precipitation of acute hyperkalemia.[8] This is a greater risk in patients with renal failure. A recent study has found no electrocardiogram (ECG) abnormalities in a number of patients, without significant renal dysfunction, treated over 1 hour.[11] The usual dose is 30–50 mg/day intravenously. This can be given three times per week for chronic therapy and is commonly given at 1 mg/kg/wk for suppression therapy in patients with AIDS. Dosing may be different in children in whom blood levels are lower.[12]

The toxicities of amphotericin B include fever, chills, rigors, nausea, vomiting, headache, anemia, and renal failure, manifested initially by hypokalemia and alkalosis, and later by decreased glomerular filtration. The fever and rigors may be a consequence of tumor necrosis factor and/or interleukin-1 release, while the anemia is caused by depression of erythropoietin.[13] Renal failure is thought to be caused in part by damage to distal tubular function[14–16] (electrolyte abnormalities due to renal tubular acidosis) and glomerulotubular flow imbalance (decreased GFR). Thrombophlebitis and local inflammation of perfused tissues or the meninges also follow administration of this highly irritating drug.

Prevention of toxicities of amphotericin B is a major aspect of treatment with this agent. The fever, chills, and gastrointestinal reactions may be ameliorated by pretreatment with antihistamine, acetaminophen, or meperidine. Treatment with erythropoietin may relieve anemia.[13] Salt loading, either with intravenous sodium-containing fluids (1,000 mL isotonic NaCl with each dose), or with a high dietary salt intake, may delay the development of renal failure.[17,18] Potassium and bicarbonate replacement may be needed to balance losses due to tubular dysfunction. Amelioration of the toxicity of intrathecal amphotericin B may be accomplished in part by the instillation of methylprednisolone (5–20 mg concurrently with the amphotericin B dose); this delays but does not prevent the ultimate development of arachnoiditis.

Given so many problems associated with administration of amphotericin B, it is not surprising that a number of efforts have been made to prevent them. There have been three approaches in an effort to reduce the dose, the first of which is administration of amphotericin B with other antifungal agents. The addition of flucytosine (100–150 mg/kg/day orally)[19] has been successfully used to reduce the dose of amphotericin B from 1 mg/kg/day to 0.3 mg/kg/day for cryptococcal meningitis in nonAIDS patients. Other ef-

Salt loading, either with intravenous sodium-containing fluids or with a high dietary salt intake, may delay the development of renal failure.

The addition of flucytosine (100–150 mg/kg/day orally) has been successfully used to reduce the dose of amphotericin B from 1 mg/kg/day to 0.3 mg/kg/day for cryptococcal meningitis in non-AIDS patients.

forts to combine amphotericin B with rifampin or other antibiotics have looked good in animal models but have not been demonstratably superior to amphotericin B alone in man.[20,21]

The second approach to lessening amphotericin B toxicity, particularly nephrotoxicity, has been to modify the molecule. Several false starts have occurred, but there are now new modified polyenes in clinical trials.

The final approach, which is now being carried into clinical trials, is the "repackaging" of amphotericin B into lipid particle vehicles. These may be liposomes, which are single or multilamellar lipid membranes enclosing an aqueous core. The amphotericin B is placed in the lipid membranes. The particles may act in part by targeting the drug to macrophages and sites of inflammation.[22] Attachment of fungal antibodies to the liposomes may further enhance targeting.[23] At present, there is clear evidence of decreased acute infusion-related toxicities, and renal dysfunction appears to be ameliorated by these agents, as does anemia. Ampholiposomes (Vestar) or in a more solid lipid particulate form, amphotericin B lipid complex (Bristol Myers-Squibb), have been used successfully for treatment of aspergillosis and hepatosplenic candidiasis in immunosuppressed patients and cutaneous leishmaniasis in Peru, and are now in early trials in coccidioidomycosis and cryptococcosis, the latter in AIDS patients.[24–28] While very promising, the utility of these lipid vehicle preparations has not been fully established.

Flucytosine

Flucytosine (5-fluorocytosine) is the sole member of the second major class of antifungals, the antimetabolites.[29] After active incorporation into the fungal cell, flucytosine is converted into 5-fluorouracil and acts as that agent. The specificity for fungi derives from the necessary conversion to the toxic drug within the fungal cell. Flucytosine theoretically is nontoxic for mammalian cells, but patients treated with flucytosine have detectable concentrations of 5-fluorouracil in their blood.[30] The origin of this, possibly conversion within the gut, is unclear.[31] High serum concentrations do not directly predict flucytosine toxicity, though they are associated with it. The spectrum of flucytosine is narrow, including *C neoformans*, *Candida* species, *Aspergillus* species, *Torulopsis glabrata*, and agents causing chromomycosis. Resistance emerges readily from multiple mechanisms, including blocks in absorption of the drug, conversion of the drug to 5-fluorouracil, and resistance to 5-fluorouracil.[32–34] In part because of the rapid emergence of resistance, flucytosine has been used primarily in combination with amphotericin B, with which it forms an additive or synergistic combination.

Unfortunately, because amphotericin B is nephrotoxic, and because flucytosine is excreted largely by the renal route, drug toxicity is a major problem when both drugs are used together. Toxicity appears after a week or more of therapy, and may be lethal. Because of myelotoxicity, flucytosine is generally used in doses of 100–150 mg/kg/day in nonleukopenic people with normal renal function, and the serum concentration should be held at about 100 μg/mL.[19] In AIDS patients the dose is commonly adjusted downward to 75–100 mg/kg/day to minimize myelotoxicity. Hepatotoxicity is also a problem, though relatively uncommon.

Flucytosine is rapidly absorbed after an oral dose and distributed well to all tissues, including the central nervous system and the cerebrospinal fluid. An intravenous form can be obtained, and the dosing is the same as for the oral form.

Azoles

The inhibition of membrane synthesis and loss of stereochemical integrity thus far appear to be reversible, and all of the agents developed thus far are fungistatic.

The antifungal azoles all act primarily by interference with electron transfer at the iron nucleus of the heme ring in cytochrome p-450.[35] The inhibition thus far appears to be reversible, and all of the agents developed are fungistatic. The drugs are relatively specific to fungal enzymes, and the consequence of this inhibition is the block of ^{14}C demethylation of lanosterol to form ergosterol. Ergosterol is the critical sterol for fungal cell membranes. Effects of azoles on the cell membranes thus include inhibition of synthesis of new membrane and loss of stereochemical integrity. Consequently, a number of membrane-associated enzymes, including those responsible for phospholipid metabolism, catalase, and peroxidase, are affected. This mechanism of action is the key to the selective activity of azoles and to some of their problems.

The first azole successfully introduced for systemic use was miconazole (Janssen Pharmaceutica, Beerse, Belgium).[36–38] This is still available (Monistat IV) and is effective against *Candida* species.[39] However, this compound suffers from the relatively poor aqueous solubility of azoles, and was dissolved in a Cremaphor solvent also used for anesthetic agents. Cremaphor is a potent histamine-releasing agent, and miconazole soon gained the reputation of causing intolerable itching after prolonged courses of administration. In addition, rapid administration caused shock and cardiac arrhythmias, which also were attributed to the vehicle.[40] This drug represents primarily a historical note for systemic antifungals, though it is a highly successful topical antifungal, now available over the counter.

The real breakthrough came with ketoconazole, which was the first of the antifungal azoles that could be administered orally. Ketoconazole had a broad antifungal spectrum, including *Candida* species, *Histoplasma*, *Paracoccidioides*, *Blastomyces*, *Coccidioides*, and *Cryptococcus*.[41,42] The ease of oral administration and dramatically reduced toxicity made ketoconazole an instant success. This was the first practical drug for chronic mucocutaneous candidiasis, and was effective for thrush and esophagitis, and even disseminated candidiasis.[43] Multicenter trials confirmed efficacy in histoplasmosis and blastomycosis, where ketoconazole (400 mg/day for 6 months) became the drug of choice.[43] Trials were not so successful in coccidioidomycosis, but the modest effect of ketoconazole made it an alternative to amphotericin B.[43–46]

Unfortunately, despite great success, ketoconazole was not the panacea for all mycotic infections. A number of problems appeared in spectrum, kinetics, and toxicities. Ketoconazole did not prove effective in either aspergillosis or zygomycosis, two major problems among the leukopenic population. Because of poor central nervous system penetration, very high doses (800–2,000 mg/day) were required for treatment of fungal meningitis.[47] Ketoconazole was effective in coccidioidal meningitis, but was not studied extensively in cryptococcal meningitis. The static nature of antifungal azoles was especially evident in coccidioidomycosis, where almost half of the responding patients later relapsed after the drug was stopped.[48,49] Further, ketoconazole was associated with intolerable nausea and vomiting in as many as half of the patients and severe depression of testosterone synthesis in men.[46–48] Ketoconazole clearly demonstrated that this class of drugs is not purely selective for fungal enzymes and can suppress mammalian C_{17-20} lyase, important in testosterone synthesis.[50,51] The resulting gynecomastia and loss of libido were major problems for male patients. These could be treated with testosterone replacement without loss of antifungal activity, but still presented problems.

Ketoconazole also has problems in absorption in that a highly acid intragastric environment is required for solubilization and absorption.[52] Thus, concurrent use of H2 blockers and antacids presents a problem, as well as achlorhydria caused by primary disease. This has been a major problem in AIDS patients, and is undoubtedly the reason for ketoconazole failures in treatment of candidal infections of mucosal surfaces.[53]

The ease of oral administration and dramatically reduced toxicity made ketoconazole an instant success.

Concurrent use of H2 blockers and antacids and achlorhydria caused by primary disease present a problem in absorption.

When it is absorbed well, ketoconazole can interact with other agents to alter serum concentrations. This occurs with cyclosporine, in which serum concentrations are markedly raised.[55,56] The astute clinician may take advantage of this by monitoring concentrations and using concurrent ketoconazole administration to permit marked reduction of cyclosporine dosing, a major cost-saving maneuver. Other adverse drug interactions include rifampin, phenytoin, barbiturates, and possibly isoniazid.[54–56]

The major toxicities of ketoconazole include dose-related toxicities already noted and non-dose-related toxicities. The latter may include dizziness, headache, rash, and hepatic toxicity. Hepatotoxicity has been the most widely publicized and has accounted for a few deaths in patients using this drug.[57] Up to 8% of patients may develop some abnormalities in liver enzymes, and about 1 in 10,000 patients are estimated to develop icteric hepatitis.[58] Because the most severe toxicities have occurred in patients taking low doses of ketoconazole, they have been considered not to be dose-dependent. This is still not totally clear, however, in part because many more patients are treated with lower doses (100–200 mg/day). There is a much larger population at risk than those receiving doses at or above 400 mg/day.

Despite the continuing popularity of ketoconazole, a search was under way for superior drugs even at the time it was introduced. This came to fruition in the triazole antifungal drugs, two of which are now in widespread clinical use. These include fluconazole, (Pfizer, Sandwich, England) and itraconazole (Janssen). The triazoles share markedly improved patient tolerance over ketoconazole, prolonged serum clearance, and reduced endocrine toxicities. However, they differ in a number of characteristics.

Itraconazole is a much more potent agent than ketoconazole and has an expanded spectrum, including *Sporothrix schenckii*, *Aspergillus* species, and agents causing chromomycosis and phaeohyphomycosis.[59,60] This agent is concentrated in fat-containing tissues, and clearance is slower both at high doses and after several weeks of administration.[61] Like ketoconazole, itraconazole requires some acid for absorption (R. Le Gendre, personal communication). In our experience, several spectacular failures have been associated with concurrent administration of H2 blockers and antacids. Itraconazole does not penetrate the cerebrospinal fluid in measurable concentrations, although Perfect et al. have found it highly successful in rabbit models of cryptococcal meningitis, and later it was found effective in humans with cryptococcal and coccidioididal meningi-

> *The triazoles share markedly improved patient tolerance over ketoconazole, prolonged serum clearance, and reduced endocrine toxicities.*

tis.[61–64] This may be due to higher concentration in meninges and brain tissue.

Itraconazole seems to have less gastrointestinal toxicity than ketoconazole, and less endocrine toxicity.[65] We have seen one patient with cortisol suppression caused by this drug. A number of patients have developed hypertension and/or edema, and several have developed hypokalemia while taking itraconazole in doses of 400–600 mg/day.[66] We have not noted alterations in aldosterone or other major mineralocorticoid precursors. Concurrent rifampin administration can reduce itraconazole serum concentrations to undetectable levels (J. R. Graybill, unpublished observations). Concurrent administration of itraconazole sharply elevated cyclosporine levels, and a 50% dose reduction with monitoring is warranted.[67]

Itraconazole is highly effective in histoplasmosis, sporotrichosis, blastomycosis, coccidioidomycosis, and paracoccidioidomycosis, and is likely to be the drug of choice in the United States the day that it is licensed.[68–71] A dose of 400 mg/day for 6 months is recommended.

Itraconazole is highly effective in vitro against *Aspergillus* species, and a small but growing experience in humans suggests great potential here.[60,62,72] In the experience of Viviani et al., seven of nine patients with invasive disease achieved remission.[62] A major limiting feature is the inability to administer the drug parenterally.

Fluconazole is a bisfluorinated triazole that is much more water soluble than the others and does not require acid for absorption.[73] This characteristic and excellent gastrointestinal tolerance has made fluconazole very popular for treatment of candidal mucosal infections in AIDS patients. Water solubility has made fluconazole the only triazole thus far available for parenteral use. Fluconazole is also excreted by the urinary route, and dose reduction is necessary in severe renal failure. Fluconazole in doses of 200–400 mg/day has been used successfully for treatment of histoplasmosis, blastomycosis and coccidioidomycosis, though data are as yet insufficient for comparisons with other azoles.[74]

Perhaps the greatest use and greatest controversy associated with fluconazole has been derived from its use in fungal meningitis.[75,76] In coccidioidal meningitis, 10 of 15 patients responded well to fluconazole, but relapses were noted.[76] In ongoing studies fluconazole has been found quite effective in coccidioidal meningitis, with only 40% failure in 38 patients treated.[76] While these results are very exciting, the greatest potential use for fluconazole may be in cryptococcal meningitis associated with HIV infection.

Itraconazole is highly effective in histoplasmosis, sporotrichosis, blastomycosis, coccidioidomycosis, and paracoccidioidomycosis.

The greatest potential use for fluconazole may be in cryptococcal meningitis associated with HIV infection.

Fluconazole 200 mg/day has been found highly effective for management of patients with AIDS after initial treatment.[77] Triazoles have also been used for primary treatment, and their place there is far more controversial. In one study, 11 of 12 patients converted cerebrospinal fluid (CSF) cultures to negative, while in others the response was less than 50%.[78–82]

A number of other triazoles have either undergone preliminary development in vitro or, in some cases, have been carried into animal models. However, these are the only two in large trials at present, and the advantages of others remain to be defined.

New Classes of Antifungals

A variety of other compounds are under or have been under active investigation. Some, such as cilofungin, other analogues, and pradimycin, may have significant broad-spectrum potential but have not been aggressively developed.[83] Benanomycin also appears to be quite promising.[84] Others, like nikkomycin, have potent activity against chitin synthase but a narrow spectrum because only *Coccidioides imitis* has sufficient amounts of chitin (and sufficient drug activity) to make this an attractive agent.[85] Yet others, such as liriodenine, are in earlier development and of less well defined potential.[86] Nevertheless, the broad range of antifungals that is represented here suggests that if major fungal pathogens are able to develop resistance to the azoles and polyenes (very minimal problems as of the present time), other alternatives will become available. Perhaps most important, despite the variety of compounds now under study, there has yet to be defined the "penicillin" of antifungals, that is, a drug that acts irreversibly and highly specifically to cause a lethal wound in the target fungal species with minimal to no adverse host effects.

Immunomodulators

A final general consideration in classes of antifungal drugs is the indirect antifungal activity of agents that ameliorate the host defect predisposing to fungal infection. They may also augment the effects of antifungals.[87–89] The most clear-cut of these is granulocyte stimulation factor, which can be used to shorten the period of severe leukopenia that follows cytotoxic therapy and, presumably, to reduce the time of vulnerability to both bacterial and fungal infections. Other agents, such as interferon gamma and tumor necrosis factor, have been suggested in animals to have a role in host defense against histoplasmosis.[90] Perhaps treatment with these agents may be useful in humans. There are major problems in our clumsy efforts to mimic nature's precise orchestration of immune responses with multiple mediators. It may be that multiple cytokines, administered together or in sequence, perhaps with vehicles that target them to specific cells, will be successful, but this is now, and will be for some time, in the realm of speculation.

MANAGEMENT OF SPECIFIC SYSTEMIC MYCOSES: 1991

One approach to the systemic mycoses is to group them by species, and another is to group them under the host immune defects that they exploit. The latter approach is used here because, although the physician treating a patient often suspects a fungal pathogen, he or she does not have an identified fungal pathogen at the time of initiation of treatment; thus a specific spectrum of likely malefactors may be chosen depending on the clinical circumstances.

Defects in Polymorphonuclear Leukocytes

The primary pathogens that cause systemic mycoses in leukopenic patients are candida, aspergillus, and zygomycetes (formerly mucor) species. Recently, *Fusarium* species and *Trichosporon beigelii* have become appreciated as important pathogens, and others less common are continually appearing in scattered reports (ie, *Blastoschizomyces capitatus*). These fungal pathogens share the characteristics of being common commensal organisms that need some additional boost to permit invasion. In the case of *Aspergillus* organisms and zygomycetes, which are inhaled as conidia and convert to mycelia, the necessary boost simply may be preconditioning with corticosteroids, hyperglycemia, or acidosis, all of which make the upper airway and sinus mucosa or the pulmonary alveoli a hospitable environment. In the case of *Candida* organisms, prior treatment with antimicrobials, hyperglycemia, and the presence of body catheters all combine to permit local overgrowth and bypass of the integument defense, with resultant fungemia.

Treatment for fungal infections may be considered under the approach to specific, known pathogens in patients with documented disease, empiric therapy of ill patients who are considered at increased risk of having a fungal infection, and prophylaxis of asymptomatic patients who have risk factors predicting an increased likelihood of fungal infection.

> *Recently,* **Fusarium** *species and* **Trichosporon beiglii** *have become appreciated as important pathogens.*

If a patient has confirmed disseminated candidiasis, mortality is usually in excess of 70%.

Documented Mycotic Infection Various investigators have addressed the approach to patients with severe leukopenia and candidiasis. Their results are remarkably uniform. If a patient has confirmed disseminated candidiasis, mortality is usually in excess of 70%, and intervention with amphotericin B appears futile.[91,92] These studies are historical collections, and patients who are treated are likely different from those who are not treated, but the outcome appears to be similar.[91–93] One notable exception exists: patients with hepatosplenic candidiasis, sometimes called chronic disseminated candidiasis. This illness begins during neutropenia, but is clinically manifested by fever and right upper quadrant pain after recovery from neutropenia. Prolonged amphotericin B therapy has resulted in cures of 30–70%, but the outcome is still grim.[95] Two recent therapeutic alternatives used have included liposomal amphotericin B, with most patients cured in one study,[28] and fluconazole, with five of six patients cured in a study from the University of Michigan.[96] Treatment was 400 mg/day, extended over more than 6 months. On the other hand, we have treated a patient with itraconazole for more than a year, only to see her relapse at completion of therapy.

Treatment of aspergillosis has been similarly frustrating, with risk of disease depending on prolonged granulocytopenia, and resolution of infection correlating more with recovery of the neutrophil counts than antifungal therapy.[97] A clinical scoring system has been proposed for identifying patients at high risk for disseminated aspergillosis, with presumptive therapy of patients who achieve a high-risk score. Another alternative is monitoring patients with nasal surveillance cultures, and then treating those patients who become positive for aspergillus.[98] This may be effective but is also costly. Clearly, treating patients very early has offered some advantage.[99,100] One regimen is amphotericin B, 1 mg/kg/day to a total dose of 30 mg/kg, with concurrent flucytosine 150 mg/kg/day. Because of predisposition to large volume hemoptysis, resection of pulmonary cavities is recommended.[101]

At present, aspergillosis is not considered a place for fluconazole treatment.

It is my impression that patients who have organ transplantation, particularly cardiac transplantation, develop a more lingering course leading to chronic invasive aspergillus. This manifests as pulmonary infiltrates and fevers that respond to amphotericin B, but often do not completely resolve.[102] We and others have seen patients treated successfully with itraconazole at 400 mg/day for 6 months or more.[60,62] Although treatment may be effective, patients must be able to take oral therapy and must not be receiving antacids or H2 antagonists. At present, aspergillosis is not considered a place for fluconazole treatment.

Empiric Treatment for High-risk Patients

Because of the difficulty of successfully treating neutropenic patients with documented fungal disease, Pizzo et al. conducted a watershed study of patients with neutropenia and fever refractory to antibacterial agents for 1 week.[103] Patients were randomized to empiric antifungal therapy or placebo. Of 18 patients who received amphotericin B, 1 developed fungal infection; 6 infections occurred in 32 patients who did not receive amphotericin B. This study has been confirmed by others in much longer trials.[104,105] This is now the standard approach to the febrile neutropenic patient. Many physicians do not wait a full week, but start amphotericin B after just a few days of fever refractory to antibacterials. In one study ketoconazole was found as effective as amphotericin B for empiric antifungal treatment, but infections with *Aspergillus* organisms were few and, to participate, patients had to tolerate oral therapy.[106] Also, *C tropicalis* responded poorly to ketoconazole.

Many physicians do not wait a full week, but start amphotericin B after just a few days of fever refractory to antibacterials.

Prophylaxis

If empiric treatment is good, would not prophylaxis be better to prevent systemic infections? A series of studies has been conducted, and thus far results are mixed. Oral nystatin and oral amphotericin B appear not much better than placebo when given to asymptomatic neutropenic patients.[107] Clotrimazole and ketoconazole appear to reduce gut colonization with *Candida* organisms, but there is overgrowth of *Torulopsis glabrata* in some series. The significance of this is not clear because *T glabrata* causes relatively little mortality, even in immunosuppressed patients. Other studies have found that mucosal infections are suppressed in patients treated with azoles compared with placebo or oral polyenes, but it is not clear that use of intravenous amphotericin B is reduced or mortality is affected.[108-114]

Other investigators have become specifically interested in prophylaxis of *Aspergillus* and have taken advantage of the initial colonization of upper-airway mucosa. Nasal sprays or even aerosols of amphotericin B have shown good effect in preventing aspergillosis in animal models, and preliminary results in humans are encouraging.[115,116] One historical comparison of itraconazole and ketoconazole suggested that the former might be effective in prophylaxis of aspergillosis in neutropenic patients.[110] However, absorption of the drug might be irregular, and unpublished follow-up studies have not been encouraging.

Local mucosal infection, such as thrush and esophagitis, may antedate the development of candidemia; prophylaxis can present this. Miconazole is effective, but costly, toxic, and invasive.[39]

Although treatment studies of established infections have not specifically addressed the question of prophylaxis of mucosal disease, various studies have compared various drug regimens that may have relevance for prophylaxis.[110,111] While clotrimazole is quite effective (50% response to a 2-week course of 5 troches daily), fluconazole for 2 weeks is more effective, with 80% responses. Relapses appear to be infrequent in fluconazole recipients as well.

Less Common Pathogens Agents of zygomycosis may cause sinus or pulmonary disease in patients who are leukopenic.[117,118] While surgical resection may be effective for sinus disease caused by these agents or *Aspergillus* organisms, noncavitary pulmonary disease is not a candidate for resection. Amphotericin B therapy is not often successful in pneumonia, and mortality is high. There have been no significant therapeutic developments in the past decade. Some would add flucytosine or rifampin to amphotericin B, but there is not clear evidence of effect. *Trichosporon beiglii* is another pathogen producing pulmonary or widely disseminated disease in neutropenic patients.[119] The organism is sensitive in vitro to amphotericin B, but clinical responses are very discouraging, and recovery of neutrophil counts may be the best hope. The same appears true for *Fusarium* organisms, agents that cause fungemia, black skin lesions, and widely disseminate by the hematogenous route.[120] To this end, treatment of the neutropenic patient with granulocyte stimulation factor may be useful in at least shortening the period of vulnerability to these infections, if not in actually treating the infection.

Defects in Cell-mediated Immunity

At present, almost every patient with AIDS has at least one episode of thrush or esophagitis, or commonly both, during his or her bout with this disease.[121] When these occur in the patient whose immune deficiency predominantly involves CD4 cells, the result is local infection without dissemination. However, patients who survive very long, into a phase where they become neutropenic, may develop candidemia and even invasive aspergillosis. The critical factor here is not cell-mediated immunity, but neutropenia from total marrow failure. Management is as for the neutropenic patient described previously.

While histoplasmosis, coccidioidomycosis, and cryptococcosis have been associated for years with defects of cell-mediated immunity, the first two were regarded as most commonly pathogens of "normal" hosts. In the midwestern United States histoplasmosis is appearing in up to 5% of patients with AIDS, and coccidioidomycosis is becoming just as common in AIDS patients living in Tucson, Arizona.[4,122]

Candidiasis

Mucosal candidiasis is clearly the most common fungal infection in patients with AIDS. Ketoconazole is effective in thrush and esophagitis.[123,124] However, it can cause nausea and vomiting, and may be poorly absorbed in patients with AIDS, thus requiring concurrent administration of acid and often doses of 400–600 mg/day.[52,53] Even when given this way, ketoconazole appears to be less effective than fluconazole.[126] Fluconazole at 200 mg/day has also been compared with clotrimazole in both a small study and a very large one (V. Pons, unpublished observations).[127] The clinical response to 21 weeks of treatment was about 90% in each group, but fluconazole treatment was associated more frequently with negative cultures at the completion of treatment, and also a much lower rate of posttreatment relapse (40%) than clotrimazole (70%). Fluconazole is also highly effective in candidal esophagitis associated with AIDS. Itraconazole is undergoing clinical investigation and appears effective in patients with AIDS and mucosal candidiasis, although data are few.

In addition to local therapy, fluconazole (and other systemic azoles) may be of value in prophylaxis of cryptococcosis and other systemic mycoses. A placebo-controlled trial is now underway in the AIDS Treatment Group (ACTG), and results should be available shortly.

Mucosal candidiasis is clearly the most common fungal infection in patients with AIDS.

Ketoconazole appears to be less effective than fluconazole in treating candidiasis.

Cryptococcosis

This occurs in 68% of AIDS patients, more than 90% of whom have positive serum latex cryptococcal agglutination tests (LCATs), thus permitting this relatively noninvasive test to serve as a sort of screen. Patients with cryptococcosis in the setting of AIDS usually have disseminated disease with meningitis, though other organs may be involved as well. Diagnosis is generally not difficult, but treatment is controversial.

In the initial large report by Kovacs et al., relapses were noted very frequently after treatment with amphotericin B and flucytosine was concluded.[128] A recent, carefully controlled study by Bozzette et al. found that after initial treatment with amphotericin B, only 1 of 37 patients randomized to fluconazole (200 mg/day) relapsed, while 10 of 34 randomized to placebo relapsed.[129] Eng and Zuger et al. suggested that relapses could be prevented with maintenance treatment using amphotericin B at 1 mg/kg/wk.[1,2] This standard practice was effective, but was associated with toxicity and frequent bacterial infections in patients with long-dwelling intravenous lines. Further, there was a question of whether results could be improved with fluconazole as used by Bozzette et al.[129]

The results of an MSG and ACTG study clearly support fluconazole over amphotericin B for suppression therapy.

The Mycoses Study Group (MSG) and the ACTG answered this question in a large study of patients who had been treated with at least 15 mg/kg amphotericin B and then were randomized to weekly amphotericin B or fluconazole at 200 mg/day.[77] In the initial data analysis, 98% of the patients treated with fluconazole sustained their remission, vs only 83% of patients randomized to amphotericin B maintenance treatment. This study clearly supports fluconazole over amphotericin B for suppression therapy.

The situation for primary treatment of cryptococcal meningitis is considerably less clear. The largest study was conducted by the MSG and ACTG. In this study, patients were given 1 dose of 400 mg of fluconazole and then 200 mg/day, with a provision to raise the dose if patients had not improved in 2 weeks.[78] The other regimen was amphotericin B, 0.3 mg/kg/day or more, with a minimal dose of 15 mg/kg over 6–10 weeks. Flucytosine treatment was left to the discretion of the investigator. Patients were randomized 2:1 fluconazole to amphotericin B.

The study was "intent to treat" in design, and all patients treated were evaluated for response. For a successful result, patients were required to have converted their CSF cultures to negative by 10 weeks of treatment. Those who were clinically quiescent but had positive CSF cultures were regarded as failures.

In the most recent (unpublished) analysis of the study, only 40% of patients treated with amphotericin B and 34% of those treated with fluconazole achieved remission of disease. Mortality was equal in both groups. A few more patients succumbed during the first week of treatment with fluconazole than with amphotericin B, but the difference was not statistically significant. There was some delay in conversion of CSF cultures to negative in patients treated with fluconazole as compared with amphotericin B. Reasons for the discouraging results are unclear, but may be the inclusion of more seriously ill patients, the fact that most patients were not treated with flucytosine, and the relatively low dose of amphotericin B used. Others had similar responses to fluconazole.[79–81]

In contrast to the above were the results of Larsen et al.[83] They conducted a study randomizing patients to either fluconazole 400 mg/day or amphotericin B 0.7 mg/kg/day for 1 week, followed by dosing 3 times per week plus flucytosine 150 mg/kg/day for 10 weeks. In their study 8 of 14 patients treated with fluconazole failed, vs 0 of 6 treated with amphotericin B and flucytosine. This study is marginal in the number of patients, and one failure in the amphotericin B groups would have voided the significance. Nevertheless, the superiority of amphotericin B and flucytosine in primary treatment was impressive. Also, like the MSG and ACTG studies, conversion of cultures to negative was slower in patients treated with fluconazole.

In an additional uncontrolled study, 14 AIDS patients were treated with itraconazole, 400 mg/day, for cryptococcal meningitis; 71% achieved remission.[63] In this study, patients with "quiescent clinical findings" but positive cultures were grouped as successes, and there was a minimum period necessary for "evaluability." This was therefore not an intent-to-treat study. Nevertheless, 10 patients clearly responded, making itraconazole a serious contender for treatment of cryptococcal meningitis. Viviani et al. also had an encouraging experience with itraconazole.[62]

Where does all of this leave us regarding primary therapy of cryptococcal meningitis in the setting of AIDS? Larsen is extremely conservative, favoring amphotericin B and flucytosine.[130] Because of the higher responses to amphotericin B and flucytosine,[82] the few early deaths seen with fluconazole treatment,[78] and the delayed culture conversions on fluconazole,[78,82] it is likely that future treatment will include at least a few weeks of high-dose amphotericin B or amphotericin B plus flucytosine. Suppression treatment will clearly be an azole. There is good experience with fluconazole, though it is uncertain whether other azoles may be as good or better than fluconazole.

It is likely that future treatment of cryptococcosis will include at least a few weeks of high-dose amphotericin B or amphotericin B plus flucytosine. Suppression treatment clearly will be an azole.

Which parameter of response should be studied? Mortality is the clearest end point, but with present regimens, deaths in the first 10 weeks of treatment are in the range of 20%, and very large numbers of patients would be required to identify a regimen significantly reducing mortality from this level. On the other hand, sterilization of cerebrospinal fluid is not achieved so readily in the first few weeks of treatment, and time to sterilization might be a fair parameter for comparison of both amphotericin B alone and with flucytosine, and later with azole-suppression treatment.

Finally, other approaches, such as very high dose azoles (800 mg/day fluconazole) fluconazole plus flucytosine, or amphotericin B lipid complex (ABLC), are all possible candidates for study. The attractiveness of such regimens may be more for the patient who relapses and needs something substantially different than a little more azole or amphotericin B. Regimens such as 800 mg/day fluconazole combined with 75–100 mg/kg/day flucytosine, or ABLC at 5 mg/kg/day, might be appropriate novel alternatives.

Histoplasmosis

Treatment of this infection is discussed in the chapter on histoplasmosis in this issue. I will limit the discussion here to a few of my personal feelings related to patients with HIV infections. Recently, itraconazole has been evaluated with >90% responses among patients with both pulmonary and disseminated disease.[131] (Wheat, J., unpublished observations) Fluconazole is currently in trials, being studied at doses of 200 and 400 mg/day.

In the HIV-infected patient, given the toxicity of amphotericin B, the problem of relapse (although suppression prevents this[132]), and the high bacterial infection rate associated with indwelling catheters, we began to use itraconazole at 400 mg/day for treatment of histoplasmosis in patients with AIDS.[131] Treatment was continued indefinitely, and of our first 13 patients treated, 11 responded with clearing of symptoms and signs, and the majority converted their cultures to negative.

More recently, the AIDS Clinical Treatment Groups have undertaken two protocols using itraconazole (Joseph Wheat, personal communication). More than 40 patients have been treated with an initial course of amphotericin B, 15 mg/kg total dose, and then switched to itraconazole at 400 mg/day. The median follow-up period is nearly a year, and there have been no failures thus far. Most recently, the ACTG have commenced a study of primary treatment with itraconazole at 400 mg/day. Very few patients have "failed," and it is not clear whether failures were clearly due to drug intolerance or disease progression. Therefore, itraconazole appears to be an outstanding agent for treatment of all but the most desperately ill patients with histoplasmosis. Patients with AIDS should be maintained on treatment indefinitely. I regard itraconazole at present as the drug of choice.

Coccidioidomycosis

Treatment of this infection is discussed in the chapter on coccidioidomycosis in this issue.

Blastomycosis There is little experience treating this infection in patients with HIV infection.[5] In the normal host, blastomycosis patients respond well to ketoconazole, with more than 80% cures.[133] However, responses are more rapid and in more than 90% treated with 400 mg/day itraconazole for 6 months (R. LeGendre, Janssen Pharmaceutica, unpublished data). There is a limited experience with fluconazole in which the MSG found only 7 of 15 responses to 50–100 mg/day, and very slow responses as compared with their experience with itraconazole. Higher doses have not helped (R. Bardsher, personal communication). Fluconazole thus is currently not likely to be widely utilized for blastomycosis.

Paracoccidioidomycosis   Paracoccidioidomycosis also rarely occurs in AIDS. Itraconazole now appears to be the drug of choice in paracoccidioidomycosis.[69,71]

Other Mycoses in Normal or Compromised Hosts

Phaeohyphomycosis These infections are caused by pigment-containing mycelial organisms that may appear quite similar to aspergillus but appear brown on hematoxylin and eosin-stained tissue. Infection may occur by inhalation or by local percutaneous inoculation. Target organs most commonly involved include the paranasal sinuses and orbit, the skin, the lungs, and musculoskeletal locations. These are chronic infections that may persist and expand over months. About half of the patients are immunosuppressed (commonly corticosteroids). Most appear sensitive to amphotericin B and itraconazole on in vitro testing, but more than half are refractory to amphotericin B treatment in vivo. In 17 such patients treated with itraconazole at 200–400 mg/day, we have had excellent responses in 11 patients, with successful responses ranging from stabilization of formerly progressing disease to complete resolution.[134]

Hyalophyphomycosis Of these agents, perhaps the most commonly encountered is *Pseudallescheria boydii*. Like phaeohyphomycosis, these organisms may infect by inhalation or direct inoculation. This infection is caused by a mycelial fungus that may be indistinguishable in tissues from aspergillus, but is readily identified in the laboratory. *P boydii* is characteristically resistant both in vitro and in vivo to amphotericin B. "Old" cures usually depended on resection of lesions when possible, and more recently in-

P boydii is characteristically resistant both in vitro and in vivo to amphotericin B.

travenous miconazole, ketoconazole, and itraconazole have been used.[135] Experience is limited, but the azoles appear to be curative in a number of patients.

Sporotrichosis This infection occurs in immunologically normal persons, and takes the form of either lymphocutaneous or noncutaneous disease. The latter included most commonly osteoarticular or pulmonary disease. While cutaneous sporotrichosis responds well to potassium iodide, this agent commonly causes allergic reactions, nausea, and vomiting. Amphotericin B has been used successfully in some patients with extracutaneous disease, but responses are often poor.

Restrepo et al. found a 100% response rate to 200 mg/day itraconazole for 6 months in the treatment of sporotrichosis.

Because of the above, ketoconazole has been used in sporotrichosis, with initially disappointing results in doses up to 600 mg/day.[136] Itraconazole has been more recently employed.[137,138] Reports are scattered, but in the largest single series, Restrepo et al. found a 100% response rate to 200 mg/day itraconazole for 6 months.[138] In a subsequent unpublished report, this series has more than doubled, with the same excellent results. In the United States a much more limited experience has been accumulated with more than 15 patients, half of whom had disseminated disease. Responses were excellent in most patients, with resolution in all patients with cutaneous disease and most with disseminated disease (Graybill, unpublished observations).

The experience with fluconazole is much smaller. We have had one failure at 100 mg/day, and a series of 12 patients recently reported also included low-dose failures. However, at 400 mg/day most patients responded with resolution of lesions. There is no experience with disseminated disease.[139]

References

1. Eng RHK, Bishburg E, Smith SM: Cryptococcal infections in patients with acquired immune deficiency syndrome. Am J Med 81:19, 1986

2. Zuger A, Schuster M, Simberkoff M et al: Maintenance amphotericin B for cryptococcal meningitis in the acquired immunodeficiency syndrome (AIDS). Ann Intern Med 109:592, 1988

3. Dismukes WE: Cryptococcal meningitis in patients with AIDS. J Infect Dis 157:624, 1988

4. Johnson PC, Kjardori N, Najjar AF et al: Progressive disseminated histoplasmosis in patients with the acquired immunodeficiency syndrome. Am J Med 85:152, 1988

5. Pappas PG, Pottage JC, Tapper ML et al: Blastomycosis in AIDS patients. Abstract 1166. Thirtieth Interscience Conference on Antimicrobial Agents and Chemotherapy, Atlanta, GA, 1990

6. Ryley JF: Chemotherapy of fungal disease. Springer-Verlag, Berlin, Heidelberg, New York, 1990

7. Brajtburg J, Powderly WG, Kobayashi GS, Medoff G: Amphotericin B: current understanding of mechanism of action. Antimicrob Agents Chemother 34:183, 1990

8. Craven PC, Gremillion DH: Risk factors of ventricular fibrillation during rapid amphotericin B infusion. Antimicrob Agents Chemother 27:868, 1985

9. Craven PC, Ludden TM, Drutz DJ et al: Excretion pathways of amphotericin B. J Infect Dis 140:329, 1979

10. Christiansen KJ, Bernard EM, Gold JWM, Armstrong DW: Distribution and activity of amphotericin B in humans. J Infect Dis 152:1037, 1985

11. Bowler WA, Hill HE, Weiss PJ et al: The safety of a one-hour infusion of amphotericin B documented by continuous electrocardiographic monitoring. Abstract 567. Thirtieth Interscience Conference on Antimicrobial Agents and Chemotherapy, Atlanta, GA, 1990

12. Starke JR, Mason EO, Kramer WG, Kaplan SL: Pharmacokinetics of amphotericin B in infants and children. J Infect Dis 155:766, 1987

13. Lin AC, Goldwasser E, Bernard EM, Chapman S: Amphotericin B blunts erythropoietin response in humans. J Infect Dis 161:348, 1990

14. Barton CH, Pahl M, Vaziri ND, Cesario T: Renal magnesium wasting associated with amphotericin B therapy. Am J Med 77:471, 1984

15. Patterson RM, Ackerman GL: Renal tubular acidosis due to amphotericin B toxicity. Arch Intern Med 127:241, 1971

16. Miller RP, Bates JH: Amphotericin B toxicity. Ann Intern Med 71:1089, 1969

17. Heidemann HT, Gerkens JF, Spickard WA et al: Amphotericin B nephrotoxicity in humans decreased by salt repletion. Am J Med 75:476, 1983

18. Branch RA: Prevention of amphotericin B-induced renal impairment. Arch Intern Med 148:2389, 1988

19. Dismukes WE, Cloud G, Gallis HA et al: Treatment of cryptococcal meningitis with combination amphotericin B and flucytosine for four as compared with six weeks. N Engl J Med 317:334, 1987

20. Beggs WH, Sarosi GA, Walker MI: Synergistic action of amphotericin B and rifampin against Candida species. J Infect Dis 133:206, 1976

21. Medoff G: Controversial areas in antifungal chemotherapy: short-course and combination therapy with amphotericin B. Rev Infect Dis 9:403, 1987

22. Gondal JA, Swartz RP, Rahman A: Therapeutic evaluation of free and liposome-encapsulated amphotericin B in the treatment of systemic candidiasis in mice. Antimicrob Agents Chemother 33:1544, 1989

23. Hospenthal DR, Rogers AL, Beneke ES: Effect of attachment of anticandidal antibody to the surfaces of liposomes encapsulating amphotericin B in the treatment of murine candidiasis. Antimicrob Agents Chemother 33:16, 1989

24. Lazar JT, Ksionski GE, Preiss SJ: Efficacy of AmBisome (liposomal amphotericin B) in opportunistic pulmonary mycoses. Abstract 569, Thirtieth Interscience Conference on Antimicrobial Agents and Chemotherapy, Atlanta, GA, 1990

25. Kan V, Bennet J, Amanthea M et al: Comparative safety and pharmacokinetic study of amphotericin B lipid complex (ABLC) and amphotericin B desoxycholate (AB) in healthy young male volunteers. Abstract 4. Thirtieth Interscience Conference on Antimicrobial Agents and Chemotherapy, Atlanta, GA, 1990

26. Llanos-Cunetas A, Chang J, Cieza J et al: Safety and tolerance of amphotericin B lipid complex (ABLC) vs Fungizone (AB) in patients with mucocutaneous leishmaniasis (MCL). Abstract 568, Thirtieth Interscience Conference on Antimicrobial Agents and Chemotherapy, Atlanta, GA, 1990

27. Yates RR, Allendoerfer R, Sun SH, Graybill JR: Comparison of amphotericin B lipid complex (ABLC) to amphotericin B (AmB) and Schering 39304 (SCH) in treatment of murine coccidioidal meningitis (CM). Abstract 285. Thirtieth Interscience Conference on Antimicrobial Agents and Chemotherapy, Atlanta, GA, 1990

28. Lopez-Berestein G, Bode GP, Frankel LS, Mehta K: Treatment of hepatosplenic candidiasis with liposomal amphotericin B. J Clin Oncol 5:310, 1987

29. Bennett JE: Flucytosine. Ann Intern Med 86:319, 1977

30. Diasio RB, Lakings DE, Bennett JE: Evidence for conversion of 5-fluorocytosine to 5-fluorouracil in humans. Antimicrob Agents Chemother 14:903, 1978

31. Harris BE, Manning BW, Federle TW, Diasio RR: Conversion of 5-fluorocytosine to 5-fluorouracil by human intestinal microflora. Antimicrob Agents Chemother 29:44, 1986

32. Block ER, Jennings AE, Bennett JE: 5-fluorocytosine resistance in *Cryptococcus neoformans*. Antimicrob Agents Chemother 3:649, 1973

33. Whelan WL, Kerridge D: Decreased activity of UMP pyrophosphorylase associated with resistance to 5-fluorocytosine in Candida albicans. Antimicrob Agents Chemother 26:570, 1984

34. Waldorf AR, Polak AM: Mechanisms of action of 5-fluorocytosine. Antimicrob Agents Chemother 23:79, 1983

35. Van den Bossche H: Biochemical targets for antifungal azole derivatives: hypothesis on the mode of action. p. 313. In McGinnis M (ed): Current topics in medical mycology. Springer-Verlag, Berlin, Heidelberg, New York, 1985

36. Stevens DA: Miconazole in the treatment of systemic infections. Am Rev Respir Dis 116:801, 1977

37. Morgans ME, Thomas MEM, Mackenzie DWR: Successful treatment of systemic cryptococcosis with miconazole. Br Med J 2:100, 1979

38. Jordan WM, Bodey GP, Rodriguez V et al: Miconazole treatment for fungal infections in cancer patients. AAC 16:792, 1979

39. Wingard JR, Vaughan WP, Braine HG: Prevention of fungal sepsis in patients with prolonged neutropenia: a randomized, double blind, placebo-controlled trial of intravenous miconazole. Am J Med 83:1103, 1987

40. Fainstein V, Bodey GP: Cardiorespiratory toxicity due to miconazole. Ann Intern Med 93:432, 1980

41. Van Cutsem J: The antifungal activity of ketoconazole. Am J Med 74(Suppl):9, 1983

42. Levine HB: Ketoconazole in the management of fungal disease. ADIS Press, New York, 1982

43. National Institute of Allergy and Infectious Diseases Mycoses Study Group: Treatment of blastomycosis and histoplasmosis with ketoconazole. Ann Intern Med 103:861, 1985

44. Graybill JR, Lundberg D, Donovan W et al: Treatment of coccidioidomycosis with ketoconazole: clinical and laboratory studies of 18 patients. Rev Infect Dis 2:661, 1980

45. DeFelice R, Galgiani JN, Campbell SC et al: Ketoconazole treatment of nonprimary coccidioidomycosis. Am J Med 72:681, 1982

46. Craven PC, Graybill JR, Jorgensen JH et al: High-dose ketoconazole for treatment of fungal infections of the central nervous system. Ann Intern Med 98:160, 1983

47. Galgianiu JN, Stevens DA, Graybill JR et al: Ketoconazole therapy of progressive coccidioidomycosis: comparison of 400- and 800-mg doses and observations at higher doses. Am J Med 84:603, 1988

48. Deresinksi SC, Stevens DA: Bone and joint coccidioidomycosis treated with miconazole. Am Rev Respir Dis 120:1101, 1979

49. Sugar A, Alsip S, Galgiani JN et al: Pharmacology and toxicity of high dose ketoconazole. Antimicrob Agents Chemother 31:1874, 1987

50. Pont A, Graybill JR, Craven PC et al: High dose ketoconazole therapy and adrenal and testicular dysfunction in humans. Arch Intern Med 144:2150, 1984

51. Britton H, Shebab Z, Lightner E et al: Adrenal response in children receiving high doses of ketoconazole for systemic coccidioidomycosis. J Pediatr 112:488, 1988

52. Lelawongs P, Barone JA, Colaizzi JL et al: Effect of food and gastric acidity on absorption of orally administered ketoconazole. Clin Pharmacol 7:228, 1988

53. Lake-Bakaar G, Tom W, Lake-Bakaar D et al: Gastropathy and ketoconazole malabsorption in the acquired immunodeficiency syndrome (AIDS). Ann Intern Med 109:471, 1988

54. Brass C, Galgiani JN, Blaschke TF et al: Disposition of ketoconazole, and oral antifungal, in humans. Antimicrob Agents Chemother 27:151, 1982

55. Meunier-Carpentier F, Heymans C, Snoeck R: Interaction of rifampcin with ketoconazole and Bay N7133 in normal volunteers. 23rd Interscience Conference on Antimicrobial Agents and Chemotherapy, Las Vegas, Oct 24–26, 1983

56. Engelhard D, Stutman HR, Marks MI: Interactions of ketoconazole with rifampin and isoniazid. N Engl J Med 311:1681, 1984

57. Duarte PA, Chow CC, Simmons F, Ruskin J: Fatal hepatitis associated with ketoconazole therapy. Arch Intern Med 144:1069, 1984

58. Janssen PAJ, Symoens JE: Hepatic reactions during ketoconazole treatment. Am J Med 74(Suppl):80, 1983

59. van Cutsem J, vanGerven F, Janssen PAJ: Activity of orally, topically, and parenterally administered itraconazole in the treatment of superficial and deep mycoses: animal models. Rev Infect Dis 9(Suppl):S15, 1987

60. Denning DW, Tucker RM, Hanson LH, Stevens DA: Treatment of invasive aspergillosis with itraconazole. Am J Med 86:791, 1989

61. Hardin TC, Graybill JR, Fetchik R: Pharmacokinetics of itraconazole following oral administration to normal volunteers. Antimicrob Agents Chemother 32:1310, 1988

62. Viviani MA, Tortorano AM, Langer M et al: Experience with itraconazole in cryptococcosis and aspergillosis. J Infect 18:151, 1989

63. Tucker RM, Denning DW, DuPont B: Itraconazole therapy for chronic coccidioidal meningitis. Ann Intern Med 112:108, 1990

64. Denning DW, Tucker RM, Hanson LH et al: Itraconazole therapy for cryptococcal meningitis and cryptococcosis. Arch Intern Med 149:2301, 1989

65. Phillips P, Graybill JR, Fetchick R, Dunn JF: Adrenal response to corticotropin during therapy with itraconazole. Antimicrob Agents Chemother 31:647, 1987

66. Sharkey PK, Rinaldi MG, Dunn JF et al: High dose itraconazole in the treatment of severe mycoses. Antimicrob Agents Chemother 35:707, 1991

67. Kramer MR, Marshall SE, Denning DW et al: Cyclosporine and itraconazole interaction in heart and lung transplant patients. Ann Intern Med 113:327, 1990

68. Phillips P, Fetchick R, Weisman I et al: Tolerance to and efficacy of itraconazole in treatment of systemic mycoses: preliminary results. Rev Infect Dis 9(Suppl):S87, 1987

69. Restrepo A, Gomez I, Robledo J et al: Itraconazole in the treatment of paracoccodioido-mycosis: a preliminary report. Rev Infect Dis 9(Suppl):S51, 1987

70. Restrepo A, Robledo J, Gomez I et al: Itraconazole therapy in lymphangitic and cutaneous sporotrichosis. Arch Dermatol 122:413, 1986

71. Negroni R, Koren F, Tiraboschi IN, Galimberti R: Oral treatment of paracoccidioidomycosis and histoplasmosis with itraconazole in humans. Rev Infect Dis 9(Suppl):S47, 1987

72. Vivani MA, Tortorano AM, Woestenborghs R, Cauwenborgh G: Experience with itraconazole in deep mycoses in Northern Italy. Mykosen 30:233, 1987

73. Thorpe JE, Baker N, Bromet-Petit M: Effect of oral antacid administration on the pharmaco-kinetics of oral fluconazole. Antimicrob Agents Chemother 34:2032, 1990

74. Galgiani JN: Fluconazole, a new antifungal agent. Ann Intern Med 113:177, 1990

75. Tucker RM, Galgiani JN, Denning DW et al: Treatment of coccidioidal meningitis with flu-conazole. Rev Infect Dis 12(Suppl):S380, 1990

76. Galgiani JN, Catanzaro A, Graybill JR et al: Fluconazole therapy for coccidioidomycosis. Abstract 574. Thirtieth Interscience Conference on Antimicrobial agents and Chemotherapy, Atlanta, GA, 1990

77. Powderly W, Saag M, Clouid G et al: Fluconazole (FLU) versus amphotericin B (AMB) as maintenance therapy for prevention of relapse of AIDS-associated cryptococcal meningitis. Abstract 1162, Thirtieth Interscience Conference on Antimicrobial Agents and Chemother-apy, Atlanta, GA, 1990

78. Dismukes WE, Cloud G, Thompson S et al: Fluconazole (FLU) versus amphotericin B (AMB) therapy (Rx) of acute cryptococcal meningitis. Abstract 1065. 29th Interscience Conference on Antimicrobial Agents and Chemotherapy, Atlanta, GA, 1989

79. Squires K, Rowland V, Gassyuk E et al: Fluconazole (FLU) as therapy for acute cryptococcal meningitis. Abstract 573, Thirtieth Interscience Conference on Antimicrobial Agents and Chemotherapy, Atlanta, GA, 1990

80. Pietrowski N, Buckley RM, Braffman MN, Stern JJ: Intravenous and oral fluconazole (FLU) in treatment of acute cryptococcal meningitis (CM) in AIDS. Abstract 576. Thirtieth Inter-science Conference on Antimicrobial Agents and Chemotherapy, Atlanta, GA, 1990

81. Sugar AM, Saunders C: Oral fluconazole as suppressive therapy of disseminated crypto-coccosis in patients with acquired immunodeficiency syndrome. Am J Med 85:481, 1988

82. Larsen RA, Leal ME, Chan LS: Fluconazole compared with amphotericin B plus flucytosine for cryptococcal meningitis in AIDS. Ann Intern Med 113:183, 1990

83. Swada Y, Nishio M, Hatori M et al: Pradimycisins D,E,FA-1 and FA-2, novel antifungal antibiotics. Abstract 691, Thirtieth Interscience Conference on Antimicrobial Agents and Chemotherapy, Atlanta, GA, 1990

84. Yamaguchi M, Hiritani T, Yamaguchi H: Mechanism of antifungal action of benanomycin A (ME1451). Abstract 590, Thirtieth Interscience Conference on Antimicrobial Agents and Chemotherapy, Atlanta, GA, 1990

85. Pappagianis D, Hector RF, Zimmer B: Nikkomycin-Z induced resolution of meningocerebral coccidioidomycosis. Abstract 596, Thirtieth Interscience Conference on Antimicrobial Agents and Chemotherapy, Atlanta, GA, 1990

86. Clark AM, Hufford CD, Ablordeppey SY et al: Antifungal alkaloids. Abstract 595, Thirtieth Interscience Conference on Antimicrobial Agents and Chemotherapy, Atlanta, GA, 1990

87. Smith PD, Lamerson CL, Banks SM et al: Granulocyte-macrophage colony-stimulating factor augments human monocyte fungicidal activity for Candida albicans. J Infect Dis 161:999, 1990

88. Martino P, Cassone A: Candidal endocarditis and treatment with fluconazole and granu-locyte-macrophage stimulating factor. Ann Intern Med 112:966, 1990

89. Anaissie E, LeGrand C, Elting L et al: Randomized trial of antibiotics (ab) granulocyte-macrophage colony-stimulating factor (GM-CSF) for febrile episodes in neutropenic cancer (ca) patients. Abstract 254. Thirtieth Interscience Conference on Antimicrobial Agents and Chemotherapy, Atlanta, GA, 1990

90. Smith JG, Magee DM, Williams DM, Graybill JR: Tumor necrosis factor alpha plays a role in host defense against Histoplasma capsulatum. J Infect Dis 162:1349, 1990

91. Maksymiuk AW, Thongprasert S, Hopfer R et al: Systemic candidiasis in cancer patients. Am J Med 77:20, 1984

92. Horn R, Wong B, Kiehn TE, Armstrong DE: Fungemia in a cancer hospital: changing frequency, earlier onset, and results of therapy. Rev Infect Dis 7:646, 1985

93. Haron E, Feld R, Tuffnell P et al: Hepatic candidiasis: an increasing problem in immunocompromised patients. Am J Med 83:17, 1987

94. Komshian SV, Uwaydah AK, Sobel JD, Crane LR: Fungemia caused by Candida species and *Torulopsis glabrata* in the hospitalized patient. Rev Infect Dis 11:379, 1989

95. Thaler M, Pastakia B, Shawker TH et al: Hepatic candidiasis in cancer patients: the evolving picture of the syndrome. Ann Intern Med 108:88, 1988

96. Kauffman CA, Bradley SF, Ross SC et al: Successful treatment of hepatic candidiasis with fluconazole. Abstract 577. Thirtieth Interscience Conference on Antimicrobial Agents and Chemotherapy, Atlanta, GA, 1990

97. Gershon SL, Talbot GH, Hurwitz S et al: Prolonged granulocytopenia: the major risk factor for invasive pulmonary aspergillosis in patients with acute leukemia. Ann Intern Med 100:345, 1984

98. Aisner J, Murillo J, Schimpff SC, Steere AC: Invasive aspergillosis in acute leukemia: correlation with nose cultures and antibiotic use. Ann Intern Med 90:4, 1979

99. Aisner J, Schimpff SC, Wiernik PH: Treatment of invasive aspergillosis: relation of early diagnosis and treatment to response. Ann Intern Med 86:539, 1977

100. Burch PA, Karp JE, Merz WG et al: Favorable outcome of aspergillosis in patients with acute leukemia. J Clin Oncol 5:1985, 1987

101. Panos RJ, Barr LF, Walsh TJ, Silverman HJ: Factors associated with fatal hemoptysis in cancer patients. Chest 94:1008, 1988

102. Binder RE, Faling LJ, Pugatch RD et al: Chronic necrotizing pulmonary aspergillosis: a discrete clinical entity. Medicine 61:109, 1982

103. Pizzo PA, Robichaud KJ, Gill FA, Witebsky FG: Empiric antibiotic and antifungal therapy for cancer patients with prolonged fever and granulocytopenia. Am J Med 72:101, 1982

104. Walsh TJ, Pizzo PA: Management of fungal infections in patients with neoplastic diseases. p. 399. In Ryley, EJF (ed): Chemotherapy of fungal diseases: handbook of experimental pharmacology. Vol 96. Springer-Verlag, Berlin, Heidelberg, New York, 1990

105. EORTC International antimicrobial cooperative group: Empiric antifungal therapy in febrile granulocytopenic patients. Am J Med 86:668, 1989

106. Fainstein V, Bodey GP, Elting L et al: Amphotericin B or ketoconazole therapy of fungal infections in neutropenic cancer patients. Antimicrob Agents Chemother 31:11, 1987

107. Shepp DH, Klosterman A, Siegel MS, Meyers JD: Comparative trial of ketoconazole and nystatin for prevention of fungal infection in neutropenic patients treated in a protective environment. J Infect Dis 152:1257, 1985

108. Anaissie E, Reuben A, Cunningham K, Bodey GP: Randomized trial of fluconazole (FLU) vs intravenous amphotericin B (IV-AmB) for antifungal prophylaxis in neutropenic patients with leukemia. Abstract 572. Thirtieth Interscience Conference on Antimicrobial Agents and Chemotherapy, Atlanta, GA, 1990

109. Tricot G, Joosten E, Boogaerts MA et al: Ketoconazole vs itraconazole for antifungal pro-phylaxis in patients with severe granulocytopenia: preliminary results of two nonrandomized studies. Rev Infect Dis 9(Suppl):S94, 1987

110. Meunier F, Aoun M, Janssens M et al: Comparison of the safety and efficacy of SCH39304 (2 regimens) and ketoconazole (Ke) as therapy (T) of oropharyngeal candidiasis (OC) in cancer patients. Abstract 579. Thirtieth Interscience Conference on Antimicrobial Agents and Chemotherapy, Atlanta, GA, 1990

111. Hann IM, Corrigan R, Keaney M et al: Ketoconazole versus nystatin plus amphotericin B for fungal prophylaxis in severely immunocompromised patients. Lancet 1:826, 1982

112. Meunier F, Aoun M, Gerard M: Therapy for oropharyngeal candidiasis in the immunocom-promised host: a randomized double-blind study of fluconazole versus ketoconazole. Rev Infect Dis 12(Suppl):S364, 1990

113. Rosenberg-Arska M, Dekker AW, Verhoff J: Efficacy of fluconazole (Fl) for prevention of fungal infections (FI) in comparison to amphotericin B (AmB) in granulocytopenic patients (pts). Abstract 577. Twenty Eighth Interscience Conference on Antimicrobial Agents and Chemotherapy. Los Angeles, CA, 23–26 October, 1988

114. Samonis G, Rolston K, Karl C et al: Prophylaxis of oropharyngeal candidiasis with flucon-azole. Rev Infect Dis 12(Suppl):S369, 1990

115. Niki Y, Bernard EM, Schmitt H-J et al: Pharmacokinetics of aerosol amphotericin B in rats. Antimicrob Agents Chemother 34:29, 1990

116. Meunier F, Leleux A, Gerain J et al: Prophylaxis of aspergillosis in neutropenic cancer patients with nasal spray of amphotericin B: A randomized prospective study. Abstract 1346. Twenty Seventh Interscience Conference on Antimicrobial Agents and Chemotherapy. New York, 1987

117. Meyer RD, Rosen P, Armstrong D: Phycomycosis complicating leukemia and lymphoma. Ann Intern Med 77:871, 1972

118. Lehrer RI, Howard DH, Sypherd PS et al: Mucormycosis. Ann Intern Med 93:93, 1980

119. Walsh TJ, Newman KR, Moody M et al: Trichosporonosis in patients with neoplastic disease. Medicine 65:268, 1986

120. Anaissie E, Nelson P, Beremand M et al: Fusarium caused hyalohyphomycosis: an overview. In Current Topics in Medical Mycology. Springer-Verlag, New York, (In Press)

121. Torrsander J, Morfeld-Manson L, Biberfeld G et al: Oral Candida albicans in HIV infection. Scand J Infect Dis 19:291, 1987

122. Ampel NM, Doos CL, Galgiani JN: Coccidioidomycosis (Coccy) among HIV-infected subjects: results from an ongoing prospective study. Abstract 1165, Thirtieth Interscience Conference on Antimicrobial Agents and Chemotherapy, Atlanta, GA, 1990

123. Fazio RA, Wickremesingh PC, Arsura EL: Ketoconazole treatment of Candida esophagitis: a prospective study of 12 causes. Am J Gastroenterol 78:261, 1983

124. Deschamps MM, Pape JW, Verdier RI et al: Treatment of Candida esophagitis in AIDS pa-tients. Am J Gastroenterol 83:20, 1988

125. deWitt S, Weeris D, Hermans P et al: Double-blind randomized study of oral fluconazole (F) versus ketoconazole (K) in 40 episodes of oropharyngeal candidiasis (OC) in ARC/AIDS patients. Abstract 572. Twenty Eighth Interscience Conference on Antimicrobial Agents and Chemotherapy. Los Angeles, CA, 23–26 October, 1988

126. Farrow PR, Brammer KW, Feczko JM: Fluconazole: a new treatment for oropharyngeal can-didiasis in AIDS and malignancy. Abstract 949. Twenty Seventh Interscience Conference on Antimicrobial Agents and Chemotherapy. New York, 4–7 October, 1987

127. Koletar SL, Russell JA, Fass RJ, Plouffe JF: Comparison of oral fluconazole and clotrimazole

troches as treatment for oral candidiasis in patients infected with human immunodeficiency virus. Antimicrob Agents Chemother 34:2276, 1990

128. Kovacs JS, Kovacs AA, Polis M et al: Cryptococcosis in the acquired immunodeficiency syndrome. Ann Intern Med 103:533, 1985

129. Bozzette SA, Larsen R, Chiu J et al: A placebo-controlled trial of maintenance therapy with fluconazole after treatment of cryptococcal meningitis in AIDS. N Engl J Med 324:580, 1991

130. Larsen RL: Azoles and AIDS. J Infect Dis 162:727, 1990

131. Graybill JR: Histoplasmosis in AIDS. J Infect Dis 158:623, 1988

132. McKinsey DS, Gupta MR, Riddler SA: Long-term amphotericin B therapy for disseminated histoplasmosis in patients with the acquired immunodeficiency syndrome (AIDS). Ann Intern Med 111:655, 1989

133. Bradsher RW, Rice DC, Abernathy RS: Ketoconazole therapy for endemic blastomycosis. Ann Intern Med 103:872, 1985

134. Sharkey PK, Graybill JR, Rinaldi MG et al: Itraconazole treatment of phaeohyphomycosis. J Am Acad Dermatol 23:577, 1990

135. Galgiani JN, Stevens DA, Graybill JR et al: *Pseudoallescheria boydii* infections treated with ketoconazole: clinical evaluations of seven patients and in vitro susceptibility results. Chest 86:219, 1984

136. Dismukes WE, Stamm AM, Graybill JR et al: Treatment of systemic mycoses with ketoconazole: emphasis on toxicity and clinical response in 52 patients Ann Intern Med 98:13, 1983

137. LaValle P, Suchil P, deOvando F, Reynoso S: Itraconazole in deep mycoses: preliminary experience in Mexico. Rev Infect Dis 9(Suppl):S64, 1987

138. Restrepo A, Robledo J, Gomez I et al: Itraconazole therapy in lymphangitic and cutaneous sporotrichosis. Arch Dermatol 122:413, 1986

139. Montero-Gei F, Stevens DA, Siles L: Fluconazole therapy in cutaneous and lymphangitic sporotrichosis. Abstract 575. Thirtieth Interscience Conference on Antimicrobial Agents and Chemotherapy, Atlanta, GA, 1990

COCCIDIOIDOMYCOSIS

NEIL M. AMPEL, MD

Coccidioidomycosis is traditionally thought of as a regional infection principally of the desert regions of the southwest United States. However, with the increasing attraction of this area as a tourist destination and its unprecedented population growth, coccidioidomycosis is developing an increasing national impact. Its prominence has also waxed with the recognition that *Coccidioides immitis* can act as an opportunistic pathogen in those with suppressed cellular immunity, such as patients with AIDS or patients who have recently undergone organ transplantation. Hence, all physicians in the United States should be aware of coccidioidomycosis and its manifestation.[1]

Coccidioidomycosis is a relatively new disease. Although it is closely associated with the North American Southwest, the first case was reported in Argentina in 1891 by Posadas.[2] Soon thereafter, a similar case was described in California by Rixford and Gilchrist.[3] An apparent pathogenic parasite was identified and named *Coccidioides immitis* for its resemblance to the protozoan *Coccididia* and its unmild character. Ophüls and Moffitt were the first to recognize the fungal nature of *C immitis* in 1900 when they studied a third patient, again from California.[2,3] Subsequently, the epidemiology and clinical manifestations of the disease were sketched out. In 1929, a laboratory accident in which a medical student inhaled a large inoculum of *C immitis* made it clear that coccidioidal infection could be benign. The innocuous and severe forms of the disease were further linked by Dickson, Gifford, and Smith in their studies of "valley fever" of the San Joaquin Valley.[2,3] The last 50 years have been characterized by a steady increase in our clinical knowledge of coccidioidomycosis and a more complete understanding of the immunologic response to *C immitis*. Several excellent reviews of coccidioidomycosis have been published, including a monograph by Fiese,[2] a state of the art review by Drutz and Catanzaro,[4] and a book edited by Stevens.[5] An international conference on coccidioidomycosis was held in 1984, and the results from this have been published.[6]

MYCOLOGY

C immitis is a fungus of uncertain taxonomic status.[7] It exists in two forms. In the soil, it grows as a mold with tube-

Coccidioidomycosis, traditionally thought of as a regional infection principally of the desert regions of the southwest United States, is developing an increasing national impact.

shaped hyphae divided by septae. Alternate cells within the hyphae degenerate, leaving thick-walled arthroconidia, each about 2–5 μm in length.[4] These are very easily dislodged and may become airborne, resulting in inhalation and infection by a susceptible host. Once within the host, the fungus rapidly alters its morphology and undergoes a unique transformation. The barrel-shaped arthroconidium swells into a globular form with thick walls, known as the spherule. Within the spherule develop small endospores, clusters of uninucleate cells. These are released when, due to unknown mechanisms, the spherule ruptures. Endospores are capable of developing into spherules, continuing the cycle, and propagating new areas of infection within the host.[8]

Suspected isolates of C immitis should be kept in sealed containers and manipulated only by experienced laboratory personnel using appropriate biosafety equipment.

C immitis grows readily on most microbiologic media, including blood and tryptic soy agar. Visible colonies can often be seen in as little as 3 days.[9,10] It is the mold or mycelial phase of the fungus that grows on laboratory media and, because this is the infectious form of the fungus, extreme caution must be exercised when handling any culture suspected of growing *C immitis*. Suspected isolates should be kept in sealed containers and manipulated only by experienced laboratory personnel using appropriate biosafety equipment.[11]

EPIDEMIOLOGY

Recent studies indicate that approximately 30% of the population in an endemic area has been previously infected with coccidioidomycosis.

It has been difficult to gauge fully the medical impact of coccidioidomycosis on populations at risk. At a single university health service within the endemic area, the average annual incidence of coccidioidomycosis among susceptible students was estimated to be 0.43%. Diagnosis and management constituted more than 2% of the clinic's visits, at an annual cost of more than $34,000.[12] It has been estimated that up to 100,000 individuals a year are infected by *C immitis*, most in the Southwest United States, at a cost of $5 million annually.[13] The prevalence of coccidioidomycosis has been based principally on skin-test reactivity to coccidioidal antigen. Recent studies indicate that approximately 30% of the population in an endemic area has been previously infected.[14,15] Although this may vary in different communities, it indicates that most individuals living in endemic areas are susceptible to infection with *C immitis*.

Coccidioidomycosis and its causative fungus, *C immitis*, are found only in the Western Hemisphere. In the United States, endemically acquired cases of coccidioidomycosis occur in the south central region of California, southern and central Arizona, the extreme southern tip of Nevada, southern New Mexico, and western Texas. However, this endemic area is spotty and incompletely defined. In general, areas endemic for coccidioidomycosis tend to be arid, with hot, dry summers and few winter freezes. However, regions not fitting this description may harbor the fungus. For example, cases have been acquired in Red Bluff, a community at the northern end of California's Sacramento Valley, and in tropical regions of Mexico and Central America.[16]

RISK FACTORS ASSOCIATED WITH SEVERE OR DISSEMINATED COCCIDIOIDOMYCOSIS

A large number of factors have been associated with the development of severe and disseminated coccidioidomycosis. While some of them are not fully established, it is important for the clinician to be aware of these factors since they could affect prognosis and outcome in any particular patient.

Race

Several early studies demonstrated a disproportionate number of Filipino and black men with severe disseminated coccidioidomycosis when compared to whites. The rate of severe disseminated coccidioidomycosis for those of Hispanic descent and for Native Americans in these studies was higher than whites but not as high as for Filipinos or blacks.[4,16]

One explanation for the increased susceptibility of members of certain races to more severe disease is an increased risk of environmental exposure. Sievers has argued for this view.[17] He and Fisher[18] found that rates of disseminated coccidioidomycosis among Pima and San Carlos Apaches living in the coccidioidal endemic region declined markedly over a 22-year period, although the rates of skin-test positivity to coccidioidin did not change. Based on this, they concluded that decreased exposure to dust contaminated with *C immitis* led to the lower prevalence of severe coccidioidomycosis.

Another possibility is that there is a genetic susceptibility to severe coccidioidomycosis. In 1977, a major wind storm swept *C immitis*-laden dust northward from the San Joaquin Valley. As a result, an outbreak of coccidioidomycosis occurred in Sacramento, California, an area not endemic for coccidioidomycosis. Subsequent to the storm, Flynn and coworkers[19] noted that there was nearly a 10-fold increase in the rate of disseminated coccidioidomycosis among black men than among white men. Environmental exposure was presumed to be similar for the two groups. Moreover, Johnson's review of death certificates in Arizona between the years 1959 and 1975 revealed higher mortality associated with coccidioidomycosis among blacks and Native Americans than among whites.[20] Additional studies, though not conclusive, indicate an increased incidence of disseminated disease among blacks and Asians as compared to whites.[16,21]

Animal data also support a genetic predisposition to severe coccidioidomycosis. Kirkland and Fierer[22] found that inbred strains of mice varied considerably in their resistance to intraperitoneal infection with *C immitis*. DBA/2 mice were more than 1,000 times more resistant to infection than were BALB/c mice. In subsequent work,[23] they found that the resistance pattern in BALB/c and DBA/2 mice was linked to a single dominant non-X-linked gene. They called this gene *Cms* and found it was not associated with resistance to other pathogens.

The issue of racial predisposition to severe coccidioidomycosis has been vigorously debated,[17,21,24–26] and currently the preponderance of data suggests that there are racial differences in the susceptibility for developing severe or disseminated coccidioidomycosis. Because of this, particular attention should be paid to this possibility in black, Filipino and other Asian, Hispanic, and Native American patients with coccidioidomycosis.[16,21]

The preponderance of data suggests that there are racial differences in the susceptibility for developing severe or disseminated coccidioidomycosis.

The Immunocompromised Host

Since Deresinski and Stevens reported their experience with 13 cases of coccidioidomycosis among compromised patients at the Stanford University Hospital,[27] physicians have recognized that patients with underlying immunodeficiencies have an increased risk of developing severe, disseminated coccidioidomycosis. In their study, the critical factor for developing disseminated coccidioidomycosis was the administration of chemotherapy. A similar conclusion was reached by Rutala and Smith in their study of patients with disseminated coccidioidomycosis admitted to the University of Arizona Medical Center.[28]

One group of patients that routinely receives immunosuppressive chemotherapy consists of organ transplant recipients. Not unexpectedly, they have been shown to have much higher rates of symptomatic coccidioidomycosis than do other patients. Cohen and coworkers[29] found that nearly 7% of all renal transplant recipients in a program in Tucson, Arizona, developed symptomatic coccidioidomycosis. The majority of the cases of coccidioidomycosis were disseminated. In contrast, only 1% of patients receiving maintenance hemodialysis over the same period developed symptomatic coccidioidomycosis. Many of the cases of symptomatic coccidioidomycosis among these transplantation recipients seemed to be due to reactivation, although two patients appeared to have acquired their initial coccidioidal infection after transplantation. Reactivation after transplantation may occur far outside the coccidioidal endemic area. Seltzer and colleagues[30] reported two cases of coccidioidomycosis after renal transplantation in San Francisco, while Vartivarian and coworkers[31] reported a case in a cardiac transplant recipient living in Virginia. In this latter case, the patient recalled a visit to Tucson 8 years prior to cardiac transplant. These studies indicate that, regardless of geographic area, all patients being considered for transplantation should be evaluated for the possibility of previous coccidioidomycosis, including a careful travel history, a coccidioidin skin test, and tube precipitin and complement-fixing antibody tests. Although no studies exist, I would recommend delaying transplantation if coccidioidal serologies are positive.

HIV Infection

Disseminated coccidioidomycosis has become a recognized complication of AIDS and HIV infection[10,32–39] since the association was first reported in 1984.[40] In fact, disseminated coccidioidomycosis in an HIV-infected patient is now an AIDS-defining condition.[41] We have recently reported our experience with 77 patients with concomitant HIV infection and coccidioidomycosis.[42] A variety of clinical syndromes was noted. The most common presentation was a diffuse pulmonary infiltrate seen on chest radiograph, similar in appearance to *Pneumocystis carinii* pneumonia, next most frequent was a focal pulmonary infiltrate; other patients presented with coccidioidal skin involvement, meningitis, and liver or lymph node infection. A small group of patients had positive coccidioidal serologies as the only manifestation of active coccidioidomycosis. The diagnosis among all patients was most frequently based on the identification of spherules in histologic specimens or the culture of *C immitis* from a biopsy. However, more than 80% of patients had positive coccidioidal serologies at the time of diagnosis. Complement-fixing antibody was more likely to be detected than tube-precipitin antibody. Patients with diffuse pulmonary involvement were less likely to demonstrate positive antibody tests. Poor outcome was related to low CD4 or T-helper lymphocyte count and to diffuse

Disseminated coccidioidomycosis has become a recognized complication of AIDS and HIV infection.

pulmonary involvement. A variety of therapies was administered to the 77 patients, including amphotericin B, ketoconazole, and the newer azole agents fluconazole and itraconazole, but there were no apparent differences in outcome based on these treatments. Of note, two patients developed active coccidioidomycosis while taking ketoconazole.

The extent to which coccidioidomycosis is a problem among individuals infected with HIV who are living in the coccidioidal endemic area is unknown. Moreover, it is not established whether most symptomatic disease is due to reactivation of a previous infection or to acute acquisition of coccidioidomycosis. In an attempt to answer these questions, we have been studying HIV-infected subjects in Arizona over the last 2 years.[43] To date, the rate of active coccidioidomycosis has been 5.25 cases for every 100 patients each year. Of the five subjects who have developed active coccidioidomycosis so far, all have had CD4 lymphocyte counts of <200/μL and none have had positive coccidioidin skin tests prior to the development of disease.

Pregnancy

Women who develop coccidioidomycosis during pregnancy, particularly the third trimester, are at increased risk for severe and disseminated disease.

Smale and Birsner first appreciated the increased risk of disseminated coccidioidomycosis in pregnant women,[44] and Vaughn and Ramirez estimated a rate of one case for every 1,000 pregnancies in the coccidioidal endemic area.[45] While the severity of maternal disease was agreed upon, the incidence was not, with some suggesting that symptomatic coccidioidomycosis during pregnancy was uncommon.[46] In a recent study, we identified a case of symptomatic coccidioidomycosis for approximately every 5,000 pregnancies among obstetrical hospitals in Tucson.[47] As other studies have shown, severity of disease increased with the time of gestation, with the most severe cases occurring postpartum. Hence, women who develop coccidioidomycosis during pregnancy, particularly during the third trimester, are at increased risk for severe and disseminated disease. The reasons for the increased risk of symptomatic coccidioidomycosis during pregnancy are speculative, but there is evidence for a general depression in cellular immunity during pregnancy.[48] As an alternative, Drutz and his colleagues have suggested that alterations in the production of various sex hormones during pregnancy may result in the direct stimulation of coccidioidal growth.[49,50,51] It is important to point out that the risk of coccidioidomycosis during pregnancy occurs only when the infection occurs during gestation; quiescent, asymptomatic infections acquired before pregnancy do not appear likely to reactivate.[8]

Sex

Although pregnancy represents a risk for severe coccidioidomycosis, in general, men are more likely to develop symptomatic illness than women.[16] For example, in a study of coccidioidal fungemia, 14 of the 15 patients were men,[10] and male sex was a risk factor for dissemination among renal transplantation recipients.[29] Possible explanations for this male predominance include an increased risk of environmental exposure or, as in pregnancy, an endocrinological factor. Testosterone, progesterone, and 17-β-estradiol are all capable of stimulating the growth of *C immitis* in vitro.[51]

Occupation

Based on the habitat of *C immitis*, it is not surprising that occupations which involve work with the soil are associated with an increased risk of acquiring coccidioidomycosis. Agricultural and construction workers are highly represented among patients,[16] and military personnel are also at increased risk. Intensive handling of soil in confined areas, as occurs with archaeologists, anthropologists, paleontologists, and zoologists,[16] may predispose not only to infection but to severe illness. Larsen and colleagues reported two cases of acute respiratory failure due to coccidioidomycosis occurring in archaeology students digging in southern California,[52] and epidemics of symptomatic disease among archaeology students have been reported in areas not previously known to be endemic for *C immitis*.[16]

Other Factors

Patients with diabetes do not appear to be at any greater risk for developing disseminated coccidioidomycosis, but they may have an increased chance of developing cavitary pulmonary disease.[16] Blood group B has been found more commonly associated with disseminated illness among renal transplant recipients.[29] There are no compelling data to suggest that age is a risk factor for the development of severe or disseminated coccidioidomycosis.[53,54] However, there have been several reports of severe infection among newborns. Infection has been noted as early as 5 days after birth. Symptoms are nonspecific and consist of fever and respiratory distress. Chest radiographs may show an initial focus of consolidation followed by diffuse infiltration. Aspiration of infected decidua at the time of birth is the most likely explanation for acquisition of infection.[55,56,57]

PATHOLOGENESIS AND IMMUNOLOGY

Infection with *C immitis* causes a mixed inflammatory response, consisting of an acute influx of polymorphonuclear leukocytes to the site of infection followed by a granulomatous response containing lymphocytes and macrophages. In most cases, infection is due to the inhalation of arthroconidia in disturbed, infected soil. Rarely, primary pulmonary infection can occur outside of the endemic area, through inhalation of contaminated dust coating items shipped from desert regions.[58]

Animal Studies

The immunological response to infection with *C immitis* has been extensively explored in animal models. From these studies, the evidence is compelling that cellular immunity involving T-lymphocytes and macrophages plays a critical role in controlling coccidioidomycosis. Beaman and colleagues demonstrated that resistance to *C immitis* could be transferred by spleen cells obtained from mice previously immunized against *C immitis*[59] While transfer of serum from immune mice had no effect on resistance to infection, inoculation of a population of cells enriched for T-lymphocytes from immune mice into nonimmune mice resulted in increased resistance in the recipients.[60] In other murine studies, macrophages were able to ingest but not kill coccidioidal arthroconidia and endospores.[61] However, coincubation of macrophages with immune lymphocytes or with soluble lymphocyte products, such as interferon-γ, did result in killing.[62,63]

Suppressor T-lymphocytes may play a role in allowing for the development of severe infection. Cox and coworkers examined the immunological differences between the susceptible BALB/c and the resistant DBA/2 mouse strains. The BALB/c mice were found to develop initial dermal hypersensitivity to inoculation with coccidioidal antigen, indicative of a cellular immune response. However, this response was lost after about 2 weeks.[64] Further work indicated that high levels of circulating antigen induced suppressor T-lymphocyte populations that inhibited the development of a protective immunologic response.[65]

Klemons et al. have demonstrated that both mononuclear cells and polymorphonuclear leukocytes may be important to the immune response to infection with *C immitis*. Beige mice, which have a polymorphonuclear cell defect, and congenitally athymic nude mice, which lack functionally mature T-lymphocytes, were both more susceptible to infection with *C immitis* than were their normal littermates.[66]

Human Studies

There are numerous studies of the human immunological response to infection with *C immitis*. Dermal hypersensitivity to coccidioidal antigen, a marker for cellular immune response, decreases with increasing severity of coccidioidomycosis and is associated with decreasing responsiveness of lymphocytes stimulated with coccidioidal antigen in vitro.[67–69] More recent studies have suggested that patients with severe coccidioidomycosis may have factors that suppress immune response. Brass and colleagues found that in vitro lymphocyte responses were decreased by a high concentration of antigen derived from coccidioidal endospores.[70] Moreover, Cox and Pope showed that in vitro lymphocyte responses were diminished by serum from subjects with active coccidioidomycosis. The suppression appeared to be mediated by anticoccidioidal monomeric IgG, either alone or complexed with coccidioidal antigen.[71] Catanzaro has presented data that indicate that suppressor T-lymphocytes may be responsible for the lack of immune response in some patients with disseminated coccidioidomycosis.[72]

Several studies have explored the role of effector cells on the immune response to infection with *C immitis*. Frey and Drutz[73] found that polymorphonuclear leukocytes were able to ingest and kill coccidioidal arthroconidia and endospores, but were unable to do either to spherules. Similarly, Galgiani and colleagues showed that polymorphonuclear leukocytes were able to inhibit the incorporation of cell-wall chitin precursors by arthroconidia.[74] Additionally, both polymorphonuclear leukocytes and mononuclear leukocytes were able to induce the formation of spherules from arthroconidia in vitro.[75] Petkus and Baum found that freshly isolated peripheral blood lymphocytes had the ability to inhibit the growth of young spherules and endospores. This activity paralleled that of natural killer cells.[76] We have recently reported that peripheral blood mononuclear cells are able to inhibit the growth of arthroconidia in vitro; this was independent of whether the donor was immune to coccidioidomycosis or not.[77]

Taken together, the data suggest that human resistance to coccidioidomycosis is dependent on cellular immunity and not on serum factors. Delayed dermal hypersensitivity, as reflected by a positive coccidioidal skin test, is predictive of a positive host response to infection with *C immitis*. The precise mechanisms that control *C immitis* infection are still not established. While it appears that polymorphonuclear leukocytes, natural killer cells, and monocytes are able to inhibit the fungus in vitro, how these cells act in vivo against the fungus is currently unknown and calls for further research.

CLINICAL MANIFESTATIONS

Pulmonary Disease

The majority of individuals with primary pulmonary coccidioidomycosis are entirely asymptomatic.

Coccidioidomycosis is protean in its clinical manifestations. The majority of individuals with primary pulmonary coccidioidomycosis are entirely asymptomatic, and infection is only detected through skin testing.[4] Symptomatic disease occurs in approximately 40% of individuals. Cough, fever, and chest pain represent the typical triad of pulmonary coccidioidomycosis.[78] Kerrick and colleagues have collated symptoms of coccidioidomycosis based on visits to a university student health service.[12] Fatigue was the most prominent complaint, followed by cough and chest pain. Rash, sore throat, and headache occurred in about one-fourth of patients. Chest pain alone has been observed as a presenting complaint in adolescents.[78] Although the symptoms of primary coccidioidomycosis are often nonspecific, some diagnostic clues exist.[4,79] A diffuse maculopapular erythematous rash develops in 10–30% of individuals. It usually occurs during the first few days of illness and may disappear by the time the patient seeks medical attention.[4] Another helpful manifestation is erythema nodosum or erythema multiforme, alone or in association with diffuse arthralgias. This syndrome, called "valley fever" or "desert rheumatism," occurs more frequently in white women and has been associated with a benign course.[4] Peripheral blood eosinophilia is one laboratory abnormality that suggests coccidioidomycosis. Echols and coworkers[80] noted mild blood eosinophilia in patients with primary coccidioidomycosis. More striking levels were seen in patients with disseminated infection. Tissue eosinophilia has also been reported during pulmonary coccidioidomycosis.[81]

The radiographic manifestations of coccidioidomycosis are multifarious. In Kerrick and colleagues' study,[12] 42% of chest radiographs revealed an infiltrate consistent with pneumonia, 8% exhibited a cavity, and 5% showed a nodule. Findings that are suggestive of coccidioidomycosis on chest radiograph include hilar adenopathy in association with a unilateral parenchymal infiltrate, pulmonary densities that disappear from one area and reappear in another, called "phantom" infiltrates, and very thin-walled cavities.[79,82] A distinct radiographic manifestation of pulmonary coccidioidomycosis is pyopneumothorax, presenting as a collapsed lung with pleural effusion.[83] This is usually due to the rupture of a coccidioidal cavity located next to the pleura.[84,85] Small pleural effusions are not uncommon, and massive effusions are occasionally seen.[86]

Nodules are a frequent radiographic presentation of pulmonary coccidioidomycosis.[87] They are usually single and 1–4 cm in size. By themselves, coccidioidal nodules are benign. They cause concern, however, because of their resemblance to pulmonary malignancies. In the endemic region, a reasonable approach in a patient with serologic or skin-test evidence of coccidioidomycosis is to observe such a lesion with serial chest radiographs. As an alternative, percutaneous needle biopsy can be performed.[88,89] Occasionally, thoracotomy is required to ensure that the nodule is not caused by a cancer.

Pulmonary cavities due to *C immitis* infection are usually single, thin-walled, and located in the upper lobe. About half will close spontaneously within 2 years. While most persistent coccidioidal cavities cause no signs or symptoms, several complications may ensue.[4] Occasionally, as mentioned above, a pyopneumothorax will develop as a result of rupture of the cavity into the pleural space. As well, the cavities can become secondarily infected with either bacteria or fungi, such as *Aspergillus* or even *C immitis* itself.[4,90,91] This complication is suggested by the collection of fluid or the development of a density within the cavity.[92] Finally, a cavity may erode into an adjacent blood vessel, resulting in sudden, massive hemorrhage.

Pulmonary cavities due to **C immitis** *are usually single, thin-walled, and located in the upper lobe.*

Persistent pneumonia due to *C immitis* is an uncommon but well-recognized sequelae of primary pulmonary coccidioidomycosis.[4,82,93] Patients experience symptoms of fatigue, chest pain, cough, and fever for more than 6 weeks. Sputum cultures usually grow *C immitis*, and coccidioidal serologies are generally positive.[93] Rarely, the pneumonic process can become chronic, resulting in scarring and fibrosis in a picture that resembles tuberculosis in its radiological appearance.[4]

Extrapulmonary Disease

In less than 1% of all cases of coccidioidomycosis, infection spreads beyond the lungs and thoracic cavity to result in disseminated infection. The most common sites of involvement are the skin, the musculoskeletal system, and the meninges, but virtually any organ may be involved. In general, extrapulmonary dissemination occurs relatively soon, usually within 1 year, after the initial pulmonary infection. However, patients with disseminated coccidioidomycosis usually do not recall the initial pulmonary event.[4]

The most common dermal manifestation of coccidioidomycosis is a chronic, irregular, vegetative growth or plaque, known as a verrucous granuloma. This was the presentation that led Posadas to first describe coccidioidomycosis in 1891.[2] Such lesions may occur singly or in groups and frequently appear on the face. Early on, they may resemble persistant pimples. Occasionally, skin lesions may overlie deeper sites of infection, such as subcutaneous abscesses or sites of osteomyelitis. These may present as nodules with draining sinuses. Diagnosis of all such lesions requires biopsy with histological examination or culture.[94,95]

Very rarely, cutaneous coccidioidomycosis may be acquired by direct inoculation through a contaminated object. These cases can be distinguished from disseminated coccidioidomycosis by the history of injury at the site of disease, the relatively short incubation period (1–3 weeks) between the time of injury and the appearance of the lesion, the lack of evidence of pulmonary disease, and the development of local lymphadenitis, which is uncommon in disseminated cutaneous involvement. It is of interest that patients with primary cutaneous coccidioidomycosis can develop both delayed dermal hypersensitivity and serologic responses to coccidioidal antigen. In many instances, primary cutaneous coccidioidomycosis heals spontaneously, but in some cases may persist and require antifungal therapy.[96]

Bone involvement occurs in 10–50% of patients with disseminated coccidioidomycosis.[97] The presentation is usually one of chronic pain, with occasional swelling and redness at the site. A cutaneous sinus tract, sometimes far distant from the involved bone, may appear. Under radiographic examination, bone involvement often presents as an irregular lytic lesion. Sclerosis is less commonly seen.[97,98] The patellae, the vertebrae, the bones of the wrist and hand, the bones of the ankle, and the clavicles are the most frequently involved.[98] The chronicity of osseous coccidioidomycosis is exemplified by a case report of a 26-year follow-up of a patient with coccidioidomycosis of the knee.[99] Rarely, tenosynovitis is a manifestation of disseminated coccidioidomycosis.[100] Although most patients with musculoskeletal coccidioidomycosis have detectable coccidioidal serologies, diagnosis requires biopsy and histological examination or culture for *C immitis*.

Central nervous system involvement by *C immitis* is one

of the most devastating manifestations of disseminated coccidioidomycosis. Subtle and nonspecific in its presentation, it is invariably fatal if not treated. Bouza and colleagues reviewed the clinical and laboratory manifestations of coccidioidal meningitis in 31 patients.[101] Symptoms and signs were vague and included headache, lethargy and confusion. Headaches were typically bilateral, throbbing, intense, and often accompanied by nausea and vomiting. Only one-third of the patients demonstrated signs of meningeal irritation, while cranial-nerve or focal neurological deficits were distinctly uncommon. Routine laboratory studies were not helpful. However, coccidioidal serologies were positive in all but 1 of the patients, and 17 of 27 had peripheral blood eosinophilia. Chest radiographs were abnormal in 22 of 30 patients, with the majority revealing unilateral, upper-lobe infiltrates. The cerebrospinal fluid (CSF) findings were consistent with that of a chronic meningitis. The mean white cell count was $260/\mu L$ and predominantly consisted of lymphocytes. Occasionally, the cells were preponderantly polymorphonuclear leukocytes or eosinophils. Low glucose and elevated protein levels were typical. Twenty-five of thirty patients had detectable complement-fixing antibody in the CSF. On the other hand, culture or visualization of *C immitis* in the CSF occurred in only one-third.

While meningitis is by far the most common manifestation of CNS coccidioidomycosis, other presentations may occur. Several cases of subarachnoid hemorrhage due to cranial aneurysms have been described.[102,103] Other complications include spinal cord compression due to extension of vertebral osteomyelitis[104] and spinal arachnoiditis resulting in spastic paraparesis.[105]

Miliary coccidioidomycosis is exhibited as a diffuse, reticulonodular pattern on chest radiograph, resembling the picture seen in miliary tuberculosis. This manifestation almost certainly represents acute, hematogenous dissemination of *C immitis*.[106] Fungemia is a common accompaniment.[10] Miliary coccidioidomycosis is most often seen in patients with profound immunosuppression and is particularly common in patients with AIDS.[10,32,42] In these latter cases, the radiographic picture may be virtually indistinguishable from *P carinii* pneumonia.

Several other organ systems are occasionally infected by *C immitis*. In the genitourinary system, endometriosis,[107,108] prostatitis,[109] epididymitis,[110] and fistulas from various genitourinary sites[111,112] have all been recently described. Although it has been suggested that the fungus rarely involves the gastrointestinal tract,[4] Weissman and colleagues described an instance where *C immitis*

Central nervous system involvement by C immitis *is one of the most devastating manifestations of disseminated coccidioidomycosis.*

Miliary coccidioidomycosis is exhibited as a diffuse, reticulonodular pattern on chest radiograph, resembling the picture seen in miliary tuberculosis.

peritonitis have been reported. Although it is usually asymptomatic and noted incidentally at surgery,[114–116] we have recently described it in association with peritoneal dialysis.[117]

Ocular manifestations of coccidioidomycosis may be expressed in two ways. Anterior chamber and conjunctivitis appear to represent hypersensitivity reactions to initial infection.[118] On the other hand, chorioretinal scars are probably due to dissemination of the fungus at some point in time. They are not, however, harbingers of progressive or severe disease.[119] On the otolaryngological front, coccidioidomycosis has been reported to cause stridor through involvement of the trachea and larynx,[120–122] to produce neck masses through the enlargement and suppuration of cervical lymph nodes,[123,124] and to cause subacute thyroiditis.[125]

DIAGNOSIS

Culture and Histology

Definitive diagnosis of coccidioidomycosis requires identification of the fungus either through isolation by culture or by identification in histopathological specimens.

Definitive diagnosis of coccidioidomycosis requires identification of the fungus either through isolation by culture or by identification in histopathological specimens. *C immitis* grows on most microbiological media, and visible colonies can be seen in as little as 3 days when cultivation is done at 37°C.[1] The fungus can be isolated from a variety of clinical sources, including sputum, bronchoscopy samples, lymph nodes, cerebrospinal fluid, bone marrow, bone, blood, and urine. Isolation of *C immitis* from blood usually augers a poor prognosis.[10] On the other hand, the finding of coccidioidouria, while useful in establishing the diagnosis of coccidioidomycosis, does not indicate disseminated or severe disease.[126] Conclusive identification of *C immitis* cannot be based on the visible appearance of the fungus but requires the finding of specific exoantigens.[127] Kits for detecting such antigens are commercially available.[128] As mentioned above, clinical cultures of *C immitis* represent an extreme biohazard and should be handled cautiously.

C immitis can also be detected in tissues using any of a number of histologic stains. In general, the hematoxylin-eosin, the periodic acid-Schiff, and the Gomori methenamine-silver stains are sufficient for identification of the fungus in histological sections.[11] Like other fungi, *C immitis* autofluoresces under ultraviolet light after hematoxylin-eosin staining, and this technique may be used in cases in which more routine measures have failed.[129] *C immitis* spherules may be seen in expectorated sputa or bronchoscopic washings using 20% potassium hydroxide (KOH), but a more sensitive method may be the use of the Papanicolaou stain that is commonly used for cytological examinations.[130] While the spherule stage of the fungus is typically seen in infected tissue specimens, occasionally hyphal elements of *C immitis* are found, particularly in chronic pulmonary cavitary disease.

Immunologic Tests

Because culture or histopathologic staining for *C immitis* may be difficult or time-consuming, tests that depend on the host's immunologic response to infection have assumed an important role in the diagnosis of coccidioidomycosis. These tests were pioneered more than 40 years ago by Dr. Charles E. Smith.[131] Since then, methodology has evolved, complicating nomenclature and producing confusion among clinicians not familiar with the techniques for detection of circulating antibody. Pappagianis and Zimmer have recently reviewed the uses of serum antibody assays in the diagnosis of coccidioidomycosis.[132]

In clinical practice, two major types of antibody tests are used in the diagnosis of coccidioidomycosis. The first is the tube-precipitin, or TP, test. TP antibody is probably an IgM-type immunoglobulin that is directed against a heat-stable antigen of *C immitis*. TP antibody is usually detected early during primary coccidioidal infection, but occasionally is found during reactivation or dissemination of disease. This reemergence may simply be an increase in the titer of a persistant but low TP antibody response. The major use of the TP antibody is in the diagnosis of acute coccidioidomycosis. Quantitative titers of TP antibody have not been established to have prognostic significance and, although TP antibody can be detected in the CSF, it has no defined role in the diagnosis or management of coccidioidal meningitis.[132]

Three methods exist for the identification of TP antibody. In the standard TP assay, serum is combined with coccidioidin and incubated at 35°C for up to 4 days. The presence of a precipitate at the bottom of the tube is indicative of a positive test. In most cases, precipitate will be seen within 24 hours. An immunodiffusion test, which relies on diffusion of antibody and antigen from wells in an agar plate, was developed for the detection of TP antibody (IDTP) by Huppert and Bailey.[133] This test may need to be carried out for a period of up to 96 hours to detect all positives, but it appears to be more sensitive than the standard TP assay.[132,134] The latex agglutination (LA) test is available as a commercial kit and is very rapid, but 6% or more of

In clinical practice, two major types of antibody tests are used in the diagnosis of coccidioidomycosis.

all positives may be false.[132] Therefore, a positive LA test must be confirmed by either the standard TP or the IDTP methods.

Complement-fixing (CF) antibodies are presumed to be IgG moieties. They tend to occur later in the course of disease than TP antibodies and may persist for prolonged periods. The quantitation of CF antibody titer has prognostic significance. The higher the titer, particularly at or above 1:16, the more likely that the patient has disseminated coccidioidomycosis. Hence, while the TP antibody need not be repeated once it is found to be positive, it is useful to follow the CF antibody titer over time. CF antibody is also useful in the diagnosis of coccidioidal meningitis. The finding of a titer of 1:2 or greater in the CSF strongly suggests the possibility of coccidioidal meningitis. While the Laboratory Branch complement-fixing (LBCF) test has been recommended as the standard for detecting coccidioidal CF antibody,[134] we prefer the immunodiffusion (IDCF) test developed by Huppert and Bailey.[135] Quantitation of the IDCF test has been found to be inexpensive and more accurate than standard quantitation techniques.[136]

In general, there are few false negative serum coccidioidal antibody tests. However, patients with depressed cellular immunity, such as those with organ transplants and those with AIDS,[39] may be less likely to have an antibody response than nonimmunosuppressed patients. False positive tests do occur rarely, usually in patients with histoplasmosis.[132] Many types of body fluids can be used for the detection of coccidioidal antibodies, but blood and CSF are the most diagnostically useful. In fact, it is unlikely that serosal fluid from any source will be positive if a serum sample is not.[132]

The skin test for delayed dermal hypersensitivity has little use in the diagnosis of acute coccidioidomycosis. A positive test indicates that infection has occurred but does not indicate when. A negative test does not exclude active infection.[1] The current major use of coccidioidal skin testing is for the epidemiologic evaluation of populations exposed to *C immitis*. In an individual patient, it may also have prognostic value. Loss of a positive skin test in a patient with active coccidioidomycosis may portend dissemination of disease, while development of a positive test in a patient with severe or disseminated coccidioidomycosis may indicate immunologic response and control of infection. Although coccidioidin, an antigen prepared from the mycelial form of the fungus, has been used for years, it has currently been supplanted by spherulin. The latter is more readily available and appears to be more sensitive than coccidioidin in the detection of delayed skin-test reactivity.[137,138] With either reagent, a positive test is indicated by induration of ≥ 5 mm 24 or 48 hours after placement. Some patients may develop a wheal minutes to hours after skin testing. This is probably an acute hypersensitivity response to either the antigen or the preservative and has no clinical significance.[132]

TREATMENT

Chemotherapy

Treatment of coccidioidomycosis is difficult, and the results are unpredictable. Drugs that have been effective in some cases have failed in other similar cases.[139] Fortunately, fewer than 5% of all patients with coccidioidomycosis require any therapy. Those who should be considered for treatment include: (1) patients with severe primary pulmonary coccidioidomycosis; (2) patients with increasing titers of CF antibody in the serum, especially $\geq 1:16$; (3) patients with fever, prostration, or worsening pulmonary disease lasting more than 6 weeks; (4) patients with evidence of infection disseminated beyond the thoracic cavity; and (5) patients with any type of coccidioidomycosis who have a depressed cellular immune response.[140]

The therapeutic options for the treatment of coccidioidomycosis fall into two groups: amphotericin B and azole antifungals, of which several are now available. Amphotericin B was introduced for the treatment of coccidioidomycosis in 1959. Although *C immitis* is uniformly susceptible to amphotericin B both in vitro and in animal models,[141] the efficacy of amphotericin B in humans has never been subjected to controlled evaluation, and its use has been empirically defined.[139] Although there are no supportive studies, most experienced clinicians feel that the current role of amphotericin B in the treatment of coccidioidomycosis is in those patients with acute, severe disease. With the availability of orally administered azole antifungal agents, the use of amphotericin B in patients with less severe and more chronic coccidioidomycosis is not defined. Amphotericin B must be given intravenously. The standard dose for an adult is 50 mg in 500 mL of 5% dextrose in water administered over 2–4 hours.[142] The drug has numerous adverse effects, including hypotension, pyrexia, nephrotoxicity, hypokalemia, hypomagnesemia,[143] acidosis, phlebitis, and anemia. The nephrotoxicity may be ameliorated through the vigorous use of intravenous saline repletion.

Amphotericin B has unique pharmacokinetics. Its ultimate metabolic fate is unknown, and it is not significantly

Treatment of coccidioidomycosis is difficult, and the results are unpredictable.

The therapeutic options for the treatment of coccidioidomycosis fall into two groups: amphotericin B and azole antifungals, several of which are now available.

cleared by the kidneys or the liver. Dosage adjustments for dysfunction of either organ are unnecessary. It has a slow elimination phase that lasts up to 15 days. This prolonged half-life allows for the administration of the drug on alternate days or even less frequently.[139] Because of dose-related nephrotoxicity, amphotericin B should be held when significant renal dysfunction occurs, usually at a serum creatinine of ≥3 mg/100 dL.[142] Potentially less toxic formulations of amphotericin B are now being developed in which the drug is bound to liposomes,[144,145] but these have not yet been studied in coccidioidomycosis.

Introduction of the imidazole antifungal drug ketoconazole in 1981 dramatically altered the treatment approach to coccidioidomycosis. Its oral absorption made it much more convenient than amphotericin B. However, initial studies examining the clinical efficacy of ketoconazole for the treatment of coccidioidomycosis were noncomparative, open evaluations of patients with progressive forms of infection.[146–149] Overall, the majority of patients with infiltrative pulmonary disease, soft tissue infection, or skeletal involvement improved, usually at doses of 400 mg/day. Patients with fibrocavitary pulmonary disease or meningitis tended not to respond. A later study[150] found no evidence that doses higher than 400 mg/day improved response rate. Additionally, up to one-third of the patients in this study had recurrences of disease within 9 months after ketoconazole was stopped. The efficacy of ketoconazole for certain kinds of coccidioidomycosis, including primary pulmonary coccidioidomycosis, vertebral osteomyelitis, and meningitis, has not been established. In addition, gastrointestinal absorption of ketoconazole is erratic and is decreased in patients with reduced gastric acidity, such as those with AIDS[151] or those receiving cimetidine.[152]

A multicenter study recently evaluated the pharmacology and toxicity of ketoconazole during the treatment of coccidioidomycosis.[153] One hundred sixty patients received 400–2,000 mg of ketoconazole per day. Within 24 hours after administration, serum levels were consistently above 1 µg/mL at all doses tested, well above the levels needed to inhibit C immitis in vitro. Penetration into the CSF was negligible. The most common adverse effects were nausea and vomiting (50%), gynecomastia (21%), and loss of libido (13%). Alopecia, elevated liver enzymes, pruritis, and rash were each seen in less than 10% of cases. Drug intolerance was dose-related and increased markedly at dosages ≥800 mg/day.

Ketoconazole has several properties unrelated to its antifungal activity.

Ketoconazole has several properties unrelated to its antifungal activity. It interferes with the cytochrome P-450 enzyme systems of several organs, inhibiting the production of a variety of steroid hormones.[154] With prolonged usage at high dosages, ketoconazole may result in gyne-comastia in men due to decreased gonadal testosterone production.[155,156] Moreover, chemical indications of adrenal insufficiency are common, although clinical manifestations are not.[157] Ketoconazole interacts with numerous drugs and can potentiate the activity of warfarin[158] and decrease the efficacy of isoniazid and rifampin.[159]

Fluconazole is a recently released triazole that is water-soluble and extremely well absorbed after oral administration. It lacks many of the adverse effects of ketoconazole and has substantial penetration into the CSF.[142] Indeed, fluconazole has been used successfully in the treatment of coccidioidal meningitis.[160,161] For nonmeningeal coccidioidomycosis, fluconazole appears to have efficacy similar to ketoconazole, but the optimal dosage is still not established.[161,162] Based on current data, 400 mg/day appears reasonable.

Fluconazole is a triazole that is water soluble and extremely well absorbed after oral administration.

Itraconazole is another triazole that has been tested for the treatment of coccidioidomycosis but is not yet released for use. It clearly has efficacy in cases of nonmeningeal coccidioidomycosis[163] and low toxicity.[164] Because it is not particularly water soluble and has relatively low CSF penetration, it was surprising when itraconazole was found to work in cases of coccidioidal meningitis. Itraconazole, like fluconazole, has efficacy in treating coccidioidal meningitis.[165]

The use of these two new triazoles in the therapy of coccidioidal meningitis has dramatically modified the therapy of coccidioidal meningitis. Prior to this, the only established treatment was intrathecal amphotericin B.[139] Depending on the expertise and preference of the physician, it was administered by cisternal, lumbar, or ventricular routes, the latter usually through an Ommaya reservoir. With careful management, survival in coccidioidal meningitis using intrathecal amphotericin B could be greater than 90%,[166] but often was much lower than this. Moreover, this therapy required either repeated injections into the subarachnoid space or the placement of a foreign body into one of the ventricles. It was not infrequently complicated by arachnoiditis or Ommaya reservoir infections. Although not yet approved for use, oral treatment with either fluconazole[161] or itraconazole may represent a reasonable alternative to the use of intrathecal amphotericin B.

Surgery

Surgery for the treatment of coccidioidomycosis has had an increasingly smaller place in the management of coccidioidomycosis over the years. It should be considered for patients with cavitary pulmonary disease complicated by pyopneumothorax, bronchopleural fistula, secondary infection, or persistent hemoptysis. Surgical debridement is also important in the management of coccidioidal osteomyelitis and in the diagnosis and drainage of soft-tissue coccidioidal masses.[1] Amphotericin B is often given perioperatively when surgery is performed for complications of coccidioidomycosis,[167,168] but the efficacy of this is unproven.

An important current role of surgery is in the diagnosis of coccidioidomycosis. Biopsy of suspected soft-tissue or skin lesions is often essential, since the appearance of many of these lesions is so often nonspecific. Surgical biopsy may also be needed in cases of solitary pulmonary nodules in order to exclude malignancy. In certain instances, careful clinical follow-up evaluation of patients with evidence of infection with *C immitis* may make biopsy unnecessary. Where biopsy is required, a first approach should be with percutaneous needle aspirate. Forseth and coworkers in a hospital in Phoenix, Arizona, reviewed the use of this technique in 348 patients. A diagnosis was established in 75%, and in 29% of these, the nodules were due to *C immitis*.[88] Diagnostic yield was higher using histopathologic examination rather than culture. In those instances in which needle aspirate fails to provide a diagnosis, open biopsy should be considered.

Overall Approach to Management

Given the array of therapies, some of which are not yet approved, and the multitudinous manifestations of coccidioidomycosis, it is difficult to suggest any particular treatment for coccidioidomycosis. However, I would recommend the following approach. For patients without underlying immunocompromising conditions with uncomplicated primary pneumonia, no therapy is needed. In chronic or persistent pneumonia or in patients with primary pneumonia and an underlying cellular immune deficiency, I would suggest the use of an oral azole antifungal, either ketoconazole or fluconazole, as initial therapy if the patient is clinically stable. Itraconazole, once approved, will probably be another appropriate alternative. For disease disseminated to the skin, soft tissue, or bones in a stable patient, oral azoles again would be an appropriate initial choice in a stable patient. The treatment of meningitis is more complex. Fluconazole clearly has efficacy, but the optimum dose is not established, nor is the drug approved for this indication. I would recommend entering any such patient into the Mycosis Study Group protocol examining the efficacy of fluconazole in coccidioidal meningitis (William E. Dismukes, MD, Principal Investigator, University of Alabama at Birmingham, personal communication). At this time, itraconazole is not approved and all patients must be treated through study protocols. Once oral azole drugs are initiated for any manifestation of coccidioidomycosis, cessation of therapy must be done cautiously and in recognition of the relatively high relapse rate. All patients should be monitored for clinical disease as well as for elevation in CF antibody titers for at least 1 year after discontinuing treatment. I would recommend the use of amphotericin B for any patient who is clinically unstable or who is unable, for whatever reason, to reliably take or absorb oral medications. Further, amphotericin B should be used in patients who fail to improve on oral azoles.

References

1. Ampel NM, Wieden MA, Galgiani JN: Coccidioidomycosis: clinical update. Rev Infect Dis 11:897, 1989

2. Fiese MJ: Coccidiodomycosis. Charles C. Thomas, Springfield, IL, 1958

3. Deresinski SC: History of coccidioidomycosis. p. 1. In Stevens DA (ed): Coccidioidomycosis: a text. Plenum Medical Book Company, New York, 1980

4. Drutz DJ, Catanzaro A: Coccidioidomycosis: state of the art. Parts I and II. Am Rev Respir Dis 117:559; 727, 1978

5. Stevens DA: Coccidioidomycosis: a text. Plenum Medical Book Company, New York, 1980

6. Einstein HE, Catanzaro A: Coccidioidomycosis. Proceedings of the 4th International Conference. Washington, DC: The National Foundation for Infectious Diseases, 1985

7. Zimmer BL, Pappagianis D: Taxonomic and physiologic characteristics of *Coccidioides immitis*. p. 165. In Leive L, Bonventre PF, Morello JA et al. (eds): Microbiology—1986. American Society for Microbiology, Washington, DC, 1986

8. Drutz DJ, Huppert M: Coccidioidomycosis: factors affecting the host–parasite interaction. J Infect Dis 147:372, 1983

9. Ampel NM, Wieden MA: Discrepancy between growth of *Coccidioides immitis* in bacterial blood culture media and a radiometric growth index. Diagn Microbiol Infect Dis 9:7, 1988

10. Ampel NM, Ryan KJ, Carry PJ et al: Fungemia due to *Coccidioides immitis*: an analysis of 16 episodes in 15 patients and a review of the literature. Medicine (Baltimore) 65:312, 1986

11. Sarosi GA, Armstrong D, Davies SF et al: Laboratory diagnosis of mycotic and specific fungal infections. Am Rev Respir Dis 132:1373, 1985

12. Kerrick SS, Lundergan LL, Galgiani JN: Coccidioidomycosis at a university health service. Am Rev Respir Dis 131:100, 1985

13. Stevens DA: *Coccidioides immitis*. p. 1485. In Mandell GL, Douglas RG, Bennett JE (eds): Principles and practice of infectious diseases, Second Edition. Wiley, New York, 1985

14. Dodge RR, Lebowitz MD, Barbee R, Burrows B: Estimates of *C immitis* infection by skin test reactivity in an endemic community. Am J Public Health 75:863, 1985

15. Galgiani JN: Development of dermal hypersensitivity to coccidioidal antigens associated with repeated skin testing. Am Rev Respir Dis 134:1045, 1986

16. Pappagianis D: Epidemiology of coccidioidomycosis. p. 190. In McGinnis MR (ed): Current topics in medical mycology. Springer-Verlag, New York, 1988

17. Sievers ML: Racial susceptibility to coccidioidomycosis [letter]. N Engl J Med 302:58, 1980

18. Sievers ML, Fisher JR: Decreasing incidence of disseminated coccidioidomycosis among Piman and San Carlos Apache Indians: a probable environmental basis. Chest 82:455, 1982

19. Flynn NM, Hoeprich PD, Kawachi MM et al: An unusual outbreak of windborne coccidioidomycosis. N Engl J Med 301:358, 1979

20. Johnson WM: Racial factors in coccidioidomycosis: mortality experience in Arizona: a review of the literature. Arizona Medicine 39:18, 1982

21. Drutz D: Racial susceptibility to coccidioidomycosis [letter]. N Engl J Med 302:59, 1980

22. Kirkland TN, Fierer J: Inbred mouse strains differ in resistance to lethal *Coccidioides immitis* infection. Infect Immun 40:912, 1983

23. Kirkland TN, Fierer J: Genetic control of resistance to *Coccidioides immitis*: a single gene that is expressed in spleen cells determines resistance. J Immunol 135:548, 1985

24. Drutz DJ: Urban coccidioidomycosis and histoplasmosis: Sacramento and Indianapolis [editorial]. N Engl J Med 301:381, 1979

25. Hoeprich PD: Racial susceptibility to coccidioidomycosis [letter]. N Engl J Med 302:59, 1980

26. Huppert M: Racism in coccidioidomycosis? Am Rev Respir Dis 118:797, 1978

27. Deresinski SC, Stevens DA: Coccidioidomycosis in compromised hosts: experience at Stanford University Hospital. Medicine (Baltimore) 54:377, 1974

28. Rutala PJ, Smith JW: Coccidioidomycosis in potentially compromised hosts: the effect of immunosuppressive therapy in dissemination. Am J Med Sci 275:283, 1978

29. Cohen IM, Galgiani JN, Potter D, Ogden DA: Coccidioidomycosis in renal replacement therapy. Arch Intern Med 142:489, 1982

30. Seltzer J, Broaddus VC, Jacobs R, Golden JA: Reactivation of *Coccidioides* infection. West J Med 145:96, 1986

31. Vartivarian SE, Coudron PE, Markowitz SM: Disseminated coccidioidomycosis: unusual manifestations in a cardiac transplantation patient. Am J Med 83:949, 1987

32. Bronnimann DA, Adam RD, Galgiani JN et al: Coccidioidomycosis in the acquired immunodeficiency syndrome. Ann Intern Med 106:372, 1987

33. Jarvik JG, Hesselink JR, Wiley C et al: Coccidioidomycotic brain abscess in an HIV-infected man. West J Med 149:83, 1988

34. Kovacs A, Forthal DN, Kovacs JA, Overturf GD: Dissemianted coccidioidomycosis in a patient with acquired immune deficiency syndrome. West J Med 140:447, 1984

35. Macher AM, De Vinatea ML, Koch Y et al: Case for diagnosis: AIDS. Milit Med 151:M57, 1986

36. Prichard JG, Sorotzkin RA, James RE 3d: Cutaneous manifestations of disseminated coccidioidomycosis in the acquired immunodeficiency syndrome. Cutis 39:203, 1987

37. Roberts CJ: Coccidioidomycosis in acquired immune deficiency syndrome: depressed humoral as well as cellular immunity. Am J Med 76:734, 1984

38. Weldon LC, Rhone DP, Bourassa R: Bronchoscopy specimens in adults with AIDS: comparative yields of cytology, histology and culture for diagnosis of infectious agents. Chest 98:24, 1990

39. Antoniskis D, Larsen RA, Akil B et al: Seronegative disseminated coccidioidomycosis in patients with HIV infection. AIDS Res Hum Retroviruses 4:691, 1990

40. Abrams DI, Robia M, Blumenfeld W et al: Disseminated coccidioidomycosis in AIDS [letter]. N Engl J Med 310:986, 1984

41. CDC: Revision of the CDC surveillance case definition for acquired immunodeficiency syndrome. MMWR 36:1S, 1987

42. Fish DG, Ampel NM, Galgiani JN et al: Coccidioidomycosis during human immunodeficiency virus infection: a review of 77 patients. Medicine (Baltimore) 69:384, 1990

43. Ampel NM, Dols CL, Galgiani JN: Coccidioidomycosis (Coccy) among HIV-infected subjects: results from an on-going prospective study [Abstract #1165]. 30th International Conference on Antimicrobial Agents and Chemotherapy. American Society for Microbiology, Atlanta, GA, 1990

44. Smale LE, Birsner JW: Maternal deaths from coccidioidomycosis. JAMA 140:1152, 1949

45. Vaughn JE, Ramirez H: Coccidioidomycosis as a complication of pregnancy. California Medicine 74:121, 1951

46. Catanzaro A: Pulmonary mycosis in pregnant women. Chest 86(Suppl):14, 1984

47. Wack EE, Ampel NM, Galgiani JN, Bronnimann DA: Coccidioidomycosis during pregnancy: an analysis of ten cases among 47,120 pregnancies. Chest 94:376, 1988

48. Weinberg ED: Pregnancy-associated depression of cell-mediated immunity. Rev Infect Dis 6:814, 1984

49. Powell BL, Drutz DJ, Huppert M, Sun SH: Relationship of progesterone- and estradiol-binding proteins in *Coccidioides immitis* to coccidioidal dissemination in pregnancy. Infect Immun 40:478, 1983

50. Powell BL, Drutz DJ: Identification of a high-affinity binder for estradiol and a low-affinity binder for testerone in *Coccidioides immitis*. Infect Immun 45:784, 1984

51. Drutz DJ, Huppert M, Sun SH: Human sex hormones stimulate the growth and maturation of *Coccidioides immitis*. Infect Immun 32:897, 1981

52. Larsen RA, Jacobson JA, Morris AH, Benowitz BA: Acute respiratory failure caused by primary pulmonary coccidioidomycosis: two case reports and a review of the literature. Am Rev Respir Dis 131:797, 1985

53. Kafka JA, Catanzaro A: Disseminated coccidioidomycosis in children. J Pediatr 98:355, 1981

54. Fulginiti VA: Commentary: coccidioidomycosis for all of us [editorial]. J Pediatr 98:411, 1981

55. Bernstein DI, Tipton JR, Schott SF, Cherry JD: Coccidioidomycosis in a neonate: maternal–infant transmission. J Pediatr 99:752, 1981

56. Child DD, Newell JD, Bjelland JC, Spark RP: Radiographic findings of pulmonary coccidioidomycosis in neonates and infants. AJR 145:261, 1985

57. Spark RP: Does transplacental spread of coccidioidomycosis occur? Report of a neonatal fatality and review of the literature. Arch Pathol Lab Med 105:347, 1981

58. Hedges E, Miller S: Coccidioidomycosis: office diagnosis and treatment. Am Fam Physician 41:1499, 1990

59. Beaman L, Pappagianis D, Benjamini E: Significance of T cells in resistance to experimental murine coccidioidomycosis. Infect Immun 580, 1977

60. Beaman L, Pappagianis D, Benjamini E: Mechanisms of resistance to infection with *Coccidioides immitis* in mice. Infect Immun 23:681, 1979

61. Beaman L, Benjamini EDP: Role of lymphocytes in macrophage-induced killing of *Coccidioides immitis* in vitro. Infect Immun 34:347, 1981

62. Beaman L, Benjamini E, Pappagianis D: Activation of macrophages by lymphokines: enhancement of phagosome-lysosome fusion and killing of *Coccidioides immitis*. Infect Immun 39:1201, 1983

63. Beaman L: Fungicidal activation of murine macrophages by recombinant gamma interferon. Infect Immun 55:2951, 1987

64. Cox RA, Kennell W, Boncyk L, Murphy JW: Induction and expression of cell-mediated immune responses in inbred mice infected with *Coccidioides immitis*. Infect Immun 56:13, 1988

65. Cox RA, Kennell W: Suppression of T-lymphocyte response by *Coccidioides immitis* antigen. Infect Immun 56:1424, 1988

66. Clemons KV, Leathers CR, Lee KW: Systemic *Coccidioides immitis* infection in nude and beige mice. Infect Immun 47:814, 1985

67. Cox RA, Vivas JR: Spectrum of in vivo and in vitro cell-mediated immune responses in coccidioidomycosis. Cell Immunol 31:130, 1977

68. Opelz G, Scheer MI: Cutaneous sensitivity and in vitro responsiveness of lymphocytes in patients with disseminated coccidioidomycosis. J Infect Dis 132:250, 1975

69. Catanzaro A, Spitler LE, Moser KM: Cellular immune response in coccidioidomycosis. Cell Immunol 15:360, 1975

70. Brass C, Levine HB, Stevens DA: Stimulation and suppression of cell-mediated immunity by endosporulation antigens of *Coccidioides immitis*. Infect Immun 35:431, 1982

71. Cox RA, Pope RM: Serum-mediated suppression of lymphocyte transformation responses in coccidioidomycosis. Infect Immun 55:1058, 1987

72. Catanzaro A: Suppressor cells in coccidioidomycosis. Cell Immunol 64:235, 1981

73. Frey CL, Drutz DJ: Influence of fungal surface components on the interaction of *Coccidioides immitis* with polymorphonuclear neutrophils. J Infect Dis 153:933, 1986

74. Galgiani JN, Payne CM, Jones JF: Human polymorphonuclear-leukocyte inhibition of incorporation of chitin precursors into mycelia of *Coccidioides immitis*. J Infect Dis 149:404, 1985

75. Galgiani JN, Hayden R, Payne CM: Leukocyte effects on the dimorphism of *Coccidioides immitis*. J Infect Dis 146:56, 1982

76. Petkus AF, Baum LL: Natural killer cell inhibition of young spherules and endospores of *Coccidioides immitis*. J Immunol 139:3107, 1987

77. Ampel NM, Galgiani JN: Interaction of human peripheral blood mononuclear cells with *Coccidioides immitis* arthroconidia. Cell Immunol 133:253, 1991

78. Tom PF, Long TJ, Fitzpatrick SB: Coccidioidomycosis in adolescents presenting as chest pain. J Adolesc Health Care 8:365, 1987

79. Bayer AS: Recognizing coccidioidomycosis. Am Fam Physician 22:133, 1980

80. Echols RM, Palmer DL, Long GW: Tissue eosinophilia in human coccidioidomycosis. Rev Infect Dis 4:656, 1982

81. Lombard CM, Tazelaar HD, Krasne DL: Pulmonary eonisophilia in coccidioidal infections. Chest 91:734, 1987

82. Bayer AS: Fungal pneumonias: pulmonary coccidioidal syndromes (part 1). Chest 79:575, 1981

83. Hyde L, Holman DC: Coccidioidal spontaneous pneumothorax. Ann Intern Med 47:1234, 1957

84. Edelstein G, Levitt RG: Cavitary coccidioidomycosis presenting as spontaneous pneumothorax. AJR 141:533, 1983

85. Cunningham RT, Einstein H: Coccidioidal pulmonary cavities with rupture. J Thorac Cardiovasc Surg 84:172, 1982

86. Pinckney L, Parker BR: Primary coccidioidomycosis in children presenting with massive pleural effusion. AJR 130:247, 1978

87. Case records of the Massachusetts General Hospital: Weekly clinicopathological exercises. Case 3-1980. N Engl J Med 302:218, 1980

88. Forseth J, Rohwedder JJ, Levine BE, Saubolle MA: Experience with needle biopsy for coccidioidal lung nodules. Arch Intern Med 146:319, 1986

89. Wright EM: The solitary pulmonary nodule [letter]. JAMA 244:1899, 1980

90. Thadepalli H, Salem FA, Mandal AK et al: Pulmonary mycetoma due to *Coccidioides immitis.* Chest 71:429, 1977

91. Rohatgi PK, Schmitt RG: Pulmonary coccidioidal mycetoma. Am J Med Sci 287:27, 1984

92. Bayer AS: Fungal pneumonias: pulmonary coccidioidal syndromes (part 2). Chest 79:686, 1981

93. Bayer AS, Yoshikawa TT, Guze LB: Chronic progressive coccidioidal pneumonitis. Arch Intern Med 139:536, 1979

94. Igelman JD, Smith BJ, Rosen T, Tschen JA: Persistent facial plaque. Arch Dermatol 123:937, 1987

95. Dickinson A, Tschen JA, Wolf JE Jr.: Coccidioidomycosis with cutaneous involvement. South Med J 77:1464, 1984

96. O'Brien JJ, Gilsdorf JR: Primary cutaneous coccidioidomycosis in childhood. Pediatr Infect Dis 5:485, 1986

97. McGahan JP, Graves DS, Palmer PES: Coccidioidal spondylitis. Radiology 136:5, 1980

98. Bried JM, Galgiani JN: *Coccidioides immitis* infections in bone and joints. Clin Orthop 211:235, 1986

99. Lantz B, Selakovich WG, Collins DN, Garvin KL: Coccidioidomycosis of the knee with a 26-year follow-up evaluation: a case report. Clin Orthop 234:183, 1988

100. Szabo RM, Lanzer WL, Gelberman RH, Haghighi P: Extensor tendon rupture due to *Coccidioides immitis.* Clin Orthop 194:176, 1985

101. Bouza E, Dreyer JS, Hewitt WL, Meyer RD: Coccidioidal meningitis: an analysis of thirty-one cases and a review of the literature. Medicine (Baltimore) 60:139, 1981

102. de Carvalho CA, Allen JN, Zafranis A, Yates AJ: Coccidioidal meningitis complicated by cerebral arteritis and infarction. Hum Pathol 11:293, 1980

103. Hadley MN, Martin NA, Spetzler RF, Johnson PC: Multiple intracranial aneurysms due to *Coccidioides immitis.* J Neurosurg 66:453, 1987

104. Delaney P, Niemann B: Spinal cord compression by *Coccidioides immitis* abscess. Arch Neurol 39:255, 1982

105. Winston DJ, Kurtz TO, Fleishmann J et al: Successful treatment of spinal arachnoiditis due to coccidioidomycosis. J Neurosurg 59:328, 1983

106. Goldstein E: Miliary and disseminated coccidioidomycosis. Ann Intern Med 89:365, 1978

107. Bylund DJ, Nanfro JJ, Marsh WJ: Coccidioidomycosis of the female genital tract. Arch Pathol Lab Med 110:232, 1986

108. Salgia K, Bhatia L, Rajashekaraiah KR et al: Coccidioidomycosis of the uterus. South Med J 75:614, 1982

109. Price MJ, Lewis EL, Carmalt JE: Coccidioidomycosis of prostate gland. Urology 19:653, 1982

110. Chen KTK: Coccidioidomycosis of the epididymis. J Urol 130:978, 1983

111. Dunne WMJ: Unexpected laboratory diagnosis of latent genitourinary coccidioidomycosis in a nonedemic area. Arch Pathol Lab Med 110:236, 1986

112. Kuntze JR, Herman MH, Evans SG: Genitourinary coccidioidomycosis. J Urol 140:370, 1988

113. Weissman IM, Moreno AJ, Parker AL et al: Gastrointestinal dissemiantion of coccidioidomycosis. Am J Gastroenterol 81:589, 1986

114. Chen KTK: Coccidioidal peritonitis. Am J Clin Pathol 80:514, 1983

115. Crum RB: Peritoneal coccidioidomycosis. Arch Surg 78:91, 1959

116. Ruddock JC, Hope RB: Coccidioidal peritonitis: diagnosis by peritonoscopy. JAMA 113:2954, 1939

117. Ampel NM, White JD, Varanasi UR et al: Coccidioidal peritonitis associated with continuous ambulatory peritoneal dialysis. Am J Kidney Dis 11:512, 1988

118. Rodenbiker HT, Ganley JP: Ocular coccidioidomycosis. Surv Ophthalmol 24:263, 1980

119. Rodenbiker HT, Ganley JP, Galgiani JN, Axline SG: Prevalence of chorioretinal scars associated with coccidioidomycosis. Arch Ophthalmol 99:71, 1981

120. Moskowitz PS, Sue JY, Gooding CA: Tracheal coccidioidomycosis causing upper airway obstruction in children. AJR 139:596, 1982

121. Gardner S, Seilheimer D, Catlin F et al: Supglottic coccidioidomycosis presenting with persistent stridor. Pediatrics 66:623, 1980

122. Batsakis JG: Coccidioidomycosis of the larynx. Pathology consultation. Ann Otol Rhinol Laryngol 93:528, 1984

123. Dudley JE: Coccidioidomycosis and neck mass 'single lesion' disseminated disease. Arch Otolaryngol Head Neck Surg 113:553, 1987

124. Newland Y, Komisar A: Coccidioidomycosis of the head and neck. Ear Nose Throat J 65:473, 1986

125. Loeb JM, Livermore BM, Wofsy D: Coccidioidomycosis of the thyroid. Ann Intern Med 91:409, 1979

126. DeFelice R, Wieden MA, Galgiani JN: The incidence and implications of coccidioidouria. Am Rev Respir Dis 125:49, 1982

127. Kaufman L, Standard P: Improved version of the exogantigen test for the identification of *Coccidioides immitis* and *Histoplasma capsulatum* cultures. J Clin Microbiol 8:42, 1978

128. Denys GA, Newman MA, Standard PG: Evaluation of a commercial exoantigen test system for the rapid identification of systemic fungal infections. Am J Clin Pathol 79:379, 1983

129. Graham AR: Fungal autofluorescence with ultraviolet illumination. Am J Clin Pathol 79:231, 1983

130. Warlick MA, Quan SF, Sobonya RE: Rapid diagnosis of pulmonary coccidioidomycosis: cytologic vs. potassium hydroxide preparations. Arch Intern Med 143:723, 1983

131. Smith CE, Saito MT, Beard RR et al: Serological tests in the diagnosis and prognosis of coccidioidomycosis. Am J Hygiene 52:1, 1950

132. Pappagianis D, Zimmer BL: Serology of coccidioidomycosis. Clin Microbiol Rev 3:247, 1990

133. Huppert M, Bailey JW: The use of immunodiffusion tests in coccidioidomycosis. II. An immunodiffusion test as a substitute for the tube precipitin test. Am J Clin Pathol 44:369, 1965

134. Kaufman L, Reiss E: Serodiagnosis of fungal diseases. p. 924. In Lennette EH, Balows A, Hausler WJJ, Shadomy HJ (eds): Manual of clinical microbiology, Fourth Edition. American Society for Microbiology, Washington, DC, 1985

135. Huppert M, Bailey JW: The use of immunodiffusion tests in coccidioidomycosis. I. The accuracy and reproducibility of the immunodiffusion test which correlates with complement fixation. Am J Clin Pathol 44:364, 1965

136. Wieden MA, Galgiani JN, Pappagianis D: Comparison of immunodiffusion techniques with standard complement fixation assay for quantitation of coccidioidal antibodies. J Clin Microbiol 18:529, 1983

137. Gifford J, Catanzaro A: A comparison of coccidioidin and spherulin skin testing in the diagnosis of coccidioidomycosis. Am Rev Respir Dis 124:440, 1981

138. Stevens DA, Levine HB, Deresinski SC, Blaine LJ: Spherulin in clinical coccidioidomycosis: comparison with coccidioidin. Chest 68:697, 1975

139. Drutz DJ: Amphotericin B in the treatment of coccidioidomycosis. Drugs 26:337, 1983

140. Stevens DA: Coccidioidomycosis and the indications for chemotherapy. Drugs 26:334, 1983

141. Collins MS, Pappagianis D: Uniform susceptibility of various strains of *Coccidioides immitis* to amphotericin B. Antimicrob Agents Chemother 11:1049, 1977

142. Graybill JR: Chemotherapy of the systemic mycoses. Semin Respir Med 9:207, 1987

143. Barton CH, Pahl M, Vaziri ND, Cesario T: Renal magnesium wasting associated with amphotericin B. Am J Med 77:471, 1984

144. Lopez-Berestein G, Fainstein V, Hopfer R et al: Liposomal amphotericin B for the treatment of systemic fungal infections in patients with cancer: a preliminary study. J Infect Dis 151:704, 1985

145. Tremblay C, Barza M, Fiore C, Szoka F: Efficacy of liposome-intercalated amphotericin B in the treatment of systemic candidiasis in mice. Antimicrob Agents Chemother 26:170, 1984

146. Galgiani JN: Ketoconazole in the treatment of coccidioidomycosis. Drugs 26:355, 1983

147. DeFelice R, Galgiani JN, Campbell SC et al: Ketoconazole treatment of nonprimary coccidioidomycosis: evaluation of 60 patients during 3 years of study. Am J Med 72:681, 1982

148. Ross JB, Levine B, Catanzaro A et al: Ketoconazole for treatment of chronic pulmonary coccidioidomycosis. Ann Intern Med 96:440, 1982

149. Catanzaro A, Einstein H, Levine B et al: Ketoconazole for treatment of disseminated coccidioidomycosis. Ann Intern Med 96:436, 1982

150. Galgiani JN, Stevens DA, Graybill JR et al: Ketoconazole therapy of progressive coccidioidomycosis: comparison of 400- and 800-mg doses and observations at higher doses. Am J Med 84:603, 1988

151. Lake-Bakaar G, Tom W, Lake-Bakaar D et al: Gastropathy and ketoconazole malabsorption in the acquired immunodeficiency syndrome (AIDS). Ann Intern Med 109:471, 1988

152. Van Tyle JH: Ketoconazole: mechanism of action, spectrum of activity, pharmacokinetics, drug interactions, adverse reactions and therapeutic use. Pharmacotherapy 4:343, 1984

153. Sugar AM, Alsip SG, Galgiani JN et al: Pharmacology and toxicity of high-dose ketoconazole. Antimicrob Agents Chemother 31:1874, 1987

154. Sonino N: The use of ketoconazole as an inhibitor of steroid production. N Engl J Med 317:812, 1987

155. Pont A, Williams PL, Azhar S et al: Ketoconazole blocks testosterone synthesis. Ann Intern Med 142:2137, 1982

156. DeFelice R, Johnson DG, Galgiani JN: Gynecomastia with ketoconazole. Antimicrob Agents Chemother 19:1073, 1981

157. Britton H, Shehab Z, Lightner E et al: Adrenal response in children receiving high doses of ketoconazole for systemic coccidioidomycosis. J Pediatr 112:488, 1988

158. Smith AG: Potentiation of oral anticoagulants by ketoconzaole. Br Med J 288:188, 1984

159. Engelhard D, Stutman HR, Marks MI: Interaction of ketoconazole with rifampin and isoniazid. N Engl J Med 311:1681, 1984

160. Tucker RM, Galgiani JN, Denning DW et al: Treatment of coccidioidal meningitis with fluconazole. Rev Infect Dis 12(Suppl 3):S380, 1990

161. Galgiani JN, Catanzaro A, Graybill JR et al: Fluconazole therapy for coccidioidomycosis [Abstract #574]. 30th Interscience Conference on Antimicrobial Agents and Chemotherapy. American Society for Microbiology, Atlanta, GA, 1990

162. Catanzaro A, Fierer J, Friedman PJ: Fluconazole in the treatment of persistent coccidioidomycosis. Chest 97:666, 1990

163. Graybill JR, Stevens DA, Galgiani JN et al: Itraconazole treatment of coccidioidomycosis. NAIAD Mycoses Study Group. Am J Med 89:282, 1990

164. Phillips P, Fetchick R, Weisman I et al: Tolerance to and efficacy of itraconazole in treatment of systemic mycoses: preliminary results. Rev Infect Dis 9(Suppl):S87, 1987

165. Tucker RM, Denning DW, Dupont B, Stevens DA: Itraconazole therapy for chronic coccidioidal meningitis. Ann Intern Med 112:108, 1990

166. Labadie EL, Hamilton RH: Survival improvement in coccidioidal meningitis by high-dose intrathecal amphotericin B. Arch Intern Med 146:2013, 1986

167. Hammon JWJ, Prager RL: Surgical management of fungal diseases of the chest. Surg Clin North Am 60:897, 1980

168. Salomon NW, Osborne R, Copeland JG: Surgical manifestations and results of treatment of pulmonary coccidioidomycosis. Ann Thorac Surg 30:433, 1980

HISTOPLASMOSIS

PHILIP C. JOHNSON, MD

DEFINITION

Histoplasmosis is a systemic disease caused by the fungus *Histoplasma capsulatum*. This fungus exists as a mycelial form in soil and is aerosolized and inhaled by man, where it converts to a yeast phase at body temperatures. The dual nature of the life cycle of *H capsulatum* allows classification of this fungus with other pathogenic dimorphic fungi, *Blastomyces dermatitidis*, *Paracoccidioides brasilensis*, *Sporotrix schenckii*, and *Coccidioides immitis*. In the endemic area for histoplasmosis, upwards of 80% of the population has skin-test evidence of previous infection.[1] It is estimated that histoplasmosis causes approximately 500,000 cases of infection annually.[2]

HISTORY

The history of histoplasmosis has gone full circle since the first case report in 1906.[3] Originally, histoplasmosis was thought to cause only a progressive disseminated disease. As further study ensued, it was realized that the infection was much more common than originally thought, and there was a high percentage of cases of asymptomatic infection limited to the respiratory tract. Now, with growing numbers of immunocompromised patients as a result of cancer chemotherapy, organ transplantation, and infectious disease processes such as the acquired immunodeficiency syndrome (AIDS), progressive disseminated histoplasmosis (PDH) is once again becoming a frequently recognized form of the disease.

Samuel Darling, a pathologist working in the Panama Canal zone, described three postmortem cases of histoplasmosis in two Martinique immigrants and one Chinese immigrant working in Panama.[3–5] Darling was looking, at the time, for the North American form of leishmaniasis, and although the organism he found was atypical for leishmaniasis, he felt it was protozoan in origin.[3] He chose the name *Histoplasma capsulatum* to emphasize the parasitized cell or histiocyte, the protozoan nature of the organism (plasma), and the fact that the organism was encapsulated (capsulatum).[3] We now know that *H capsulatum* is a fungus and does not contain a capsule per se, although it does infect histiocytic cells.

Riley and Watson from Minnesota described the first case of histoplasmosis in the United States in 1926.[6] The patient, a chicken farmer, died of PDH and the autopsy revealed diffuse involvement of the reticuloendothelial system. Dodd and Tompkins reported the earliest case of histoplasmosis during life in a 6-month-old infant from Nashville, Tennessee in 1934.[7] The diagnosis was made by observing the organism within mononuclear cells of a peripheral blood smear. De Monbreun cultured the organism from the same infant and showed that *H capsulatum* was a dimorphic fungus.[8] For the next 20 years, 71 cases were reported, all describing progressive disseminated disease that almost always proved fatal.[9]

This conclusion was soon challenged after a histoplasmin skin test was developed. Christi, Peterson, and Palmer performed studies showing that histoplasmin skin-test reactivity was common in asymptomatic individuals.[1,10–12] The U.S. Public Health Service conducted extensive skin-test surveys among members of the U.S. Navy, and the endemic area was mapped precisely.[1] Over 80% of Navy recruits from the Mississippi and Ohio River Valley areas showed histoplasmin skin-test reactivity.[1] The endemic area was found to extend into eastern Texas, Oklahoma, and Kansas; across the Midwest to portions of Pennsylvania, Delaware, and Virginia; and southward through the Carolinas, Georgia, and Alabama. Isolated areas of skin-test reactivity were also found in parts of Florida, Minnesota, New York, Colorado, and Nebraska. Cases of benign pulmonary histoplasmosis were soon reported once it became clear that histoplasmosis was not a uniformly fatal disseminated disease.[13]

In the 1950s it was discovered that *H capsulatum* was present in nature, found in the soil in microfoci contaminated with high concentrations of organisms.[14] These microfoci usually occur in areas where bird or bat excrement has fallen onto the soil.[15] Outbreaks associated with chicken coops, caves, attics, dead trees, and activities that disturb these microfoci were reported. Schwartz showed the relationship of splenic calcifications to histoplasmosis in an autopsy series performed in Cincinnati, Ohio.[16] From this it was postulated that, once inhaled, the organism disseminates through the body with minimal sequelae. The spleen serves as a trap for disseminated organisms.

A chronic form of pulmonary histoplasmosis was recognized in 1956.[17] Patients in a tuberculosis sanitorium were found to have culture and serologic evidence of histoplasmosis. They had been previously thought to have pulmonary tuberculosis with upper-lobe fibrocavitary infiltrates. These patients were shown to react to histoplasmin skin tests. Later, this new form of histoplasmosis was referred to as chronic pulmonary histoplasmosis and was described in patients who were primarily middle-aged and had evidence of centrilobular emphysema.[18]

The pendulum swung back to progressive disseminated disease as cytotoxic chemotherapies for malignancies and immunosuppression regimens for organ transplantations were devised. Cases of PDH were soon recognized in these patients.[19-22] Amphotericin B (AMB), the mainstay in antifungal chemotherapy, was used successfully to eradicate the infection even in these immunosuppressed hosts.

Cases of PDH were recognized late but in increasing numbers after the outbreak of the AIDS epidemic in the United States in 1981.[23-26] This is likely because the regions of the United States with early concentrations of AIDS patients were the coasts rather than the endemic area for histoplasmosis. The disease in these severely immunocompromised patients mimicked the infantile form of PDH described years earlier by Darling and others.[3-5,27] Patients with AIDS and PDH had evidence of severe parasitization of the reticuloendothelial system manifested by anemia, leukopenia, and thrombocytopenia as well as hepatomegaly, splenomegaly, and lymphadenopathy.[28] Unusual manifestations of histoplasmosis, including cutaneous involvement and cerebral involvement, and ultimately ending fatally in disseminating intravascular coagulation have been reported.[29] Treatment of this condition in persons with AIDS is difficult and requires life-long suppression with AMB.[29]

EPIDEMIOLOGY

H capsulatum is highly endemic in the southeastern and central United States along the states bordering the Mississippi and Ohio River Valleys. The overall instance of skin-test reactivity in the United States is 22%; however, in the endemic area skin-test reactivity may exceed 80%. The endemic zone continues throughout Mexico and Central America and extends to areas of South America. The Caribbean region, including the islands of Hispañola and Puerto Rico, are also endemic for *H capsulatum*. Within the endemic zone there are suspected microfoci of contaminated soil that can result in occasional outbreaks when a number of susceptible people are present.[30,31] Such microfoci have been discovered as a result of earth-moving activities for road construction and in caves when soil is disturbed during spelunking.

H capsulatum *is highly endemic in the southeastern and central United States along the states bordering the Ohio and Mississippi River Valleys.*

TABLE 1   Selected Outbreaks of Histoplasmosis

Location	Population Exposed	Attach Rate %	Site	Activity
New York	21	90	Bell tower	Shoveling pigeon droppings
Oklahoma	42	74	Storm cellar	Chopping rotten wood
Wisconsin	23	83	Blackbird roost in vacant lot	Digging sewer lines
Mississippi	33	36	Soil from blackbird roost	Tossing bag of soil around class
Ohio	949	40	Blackbird roost in courtyard	Raking leaves and sweeping dirt
Colorado	29	79	Cave	Throwing dirt at bats
Indiana	—	—	—	Felling rotten trees

Data from references 34, 36–44.

H capsulatum was first isolated from the soil in 1949.[14] Soil favoring heavy growth of *H capsulatum* usually contains a high nitrogen content as a result of contamination with bird and bat excreta. Bats have been shown to develop histoplasmosis and pass organisms in their stool.[32,33] Birds and chickens, on the other hand, are not susceptible to *H capsulatum* infection since the organism cannot survive their elevated body temperatures.[34] In these situations it is felt that the bird excreta provides nitrogen and other nutrients required for growth of the fungus. Humid conditions may also favor growth of the organism. Several outbreaks have been described occurring as a result of the felling of rotted trees and collecting of firewood. Until recently, it was suspected that these sites were contaminated with bird excreta that harbored the organism, although now it appears that rotted wood alone can support the growth of the organism much in the same way as soil.[35] Contamination with bird excreta may have facilitated growth, but was not necessary for it. This finding may explain the occurrence of isolated cases of histoplasmosis following tree-cutting operations. Table 1 shows other activities that have been related to outbreaks of histoplasmosis.

Microconidia are inhaled into the distal alveolar septa where they convert to the yeast phase at body temperatures. The yeast is carried by lymphatics and blood vessels to the reticuloendothelial system.

PATHOGENESIS

With the exception of rare cases of primary inoculation exposure that have been described in the microbiology laboratory,[45,46] histoplasmosis occurs from inhalation of microconidia from the organism's mycelial growth phase into the distal alveolar septa of the lungs. These microconidia are sufficiently small to be carried directly to the alveoli.

At body temperature in the alveoli they germinate and convert to the yeast phase of the organism, and infection begins. Growth occurs by binary fission.[47] The exact number of organisms required for infection is unknown; however, in outbreaks, the concentration of organisms appears to follow the severity of disease. People exposed to high concentrations of organisms in a small, confined space, such as a cave, usually have the most severe pulmonary symptoms, whereas those exposed to small numbers of organisms as a result of earth-moving activities in open spaces experience less severe symptoms. Person-to-person spread by droplet nuclei is not reported because the mycelial phase is required for sporulation. Only the yeast phase occurs at body temperatures.

Understanding about the host response to infection has been obtained from clinical pathologic specimens and from a murine model. Once inhaled, the organism grows locally at the site of infection in the lung parenchyma. An initial response with polymorphonuclear leukocyte infiltration of infected areas occurs and lasts during the first week after infection. Neutrophils disappear as helper-inducer lymphocytes and macrophages migrate to the tissues.[48] It is these armed macrophages that are able to halt progression of the disease, although they serve as locations of fungal growth. In vitro studies done by Shaffner and colleagues have shown that the in vitro mycelial form of *H capsulatum* is killed by neutrophils, whereas the yeast form is highly resistant to these cells.[49] This is in contradistinction to opportunistic fungi, which are readily killed by neutrophils in vitro.[49] When neutrophils encounter *H capsulatum* yeast forms, a typical respiratory burst is observed; however, the yeast phase appears less susceptible to hydrogen peroxide. During mononuclear phagocytosis, the growth of *H capsulatum* yeast forms is enhanced; this results in an exudative process that corresponds to the pneumonitis observed clinically.

Some of the fungi are carried by lymphatics and blood vessels to other cells within the reticuloendothelial system, including regional lymph nodes, liver, and spleen. In a murine model of histoplasmosis, pretreatment of helper-inducer lymphocytes with an antihelper lymphocyte monoclonal antibody resulted in a marked increase in the number of organisms in the spleen. Granuloma formation in these animals was unchanged when compared to the control group, which was not treated. However, the lack of helper-inducer lymphocytes resulted in a lethal infection in the animals treated.[50] This experiment has a correlate in immunocompromised patients exposed to histoplasmosis. In normal hosts within a period of several weeks, cell-mediated immunity occurs, producing granuloma formation in pulmonary tissues, regional lymph nodes, liver, and spleen. Concomitant with the development of cell-mediated immunity is conversion of the histoplasma skin test. Antibody tests to *H capsulatum* become positive generally 4–6 weeks after initial infection.

Over time, granulomas tend to heal by fibrosis and calcification. Since primary pulmonary disease is usually asymptomatic, these calcified granulomas are later observed on normal chest roentgenograms as calcifications in the lung and spleen of patients previously exposed to histoplasmosis. Over a period of years, cell-mediated immunity to the organism may wane, especially in situations in which repetitive exposure does not occur. Reinfection may occur in this setting, with resultant stimulation of cell-mediated and humoral immunity to the organism. Goodwin and colleagues have shown that this occurrence can modify the clinical course of infection.[34] Individuals with waning immunity to *H capsulatum* become symptomatic only after a high exposure, whereas their naive counterparts can experience illness after exposure to microfoci with relatively few organisms. The symptoms of those with previous exposure usually occur earlier than those of patients who have not been exposed, and these symptoms are not as severe.

Over the last 20 years, the effect of cancer chemotherapy, treatment to prevent transplanted organ rejection, and infection with HIV have resulted in a group of immunosuppressed individuals who have increased susceptibility to *H capsulatum* infection and to reactivation of past disease. The role primary exposure and reactivation of previous infection might play in the pathogenesis of disease in these patients is unclear. Among patients with AIDS and PDH in Houston, Texas, an area on the fringes of the endemic zone, we have speculated that reactivation is the primary cause of disease.[28] Among patients with AIDS described in Indianapolis, Indiana, a city that has recently experienced several large outbreaks of histoplasmosis, PDH appears to result from either primary infection or reinfection in patients whose immunity has waned.[44,51] Evidence for reactivation is a paucity of pulmonary findings in at least one-half of the patients from the Houston series[29] and the description of cases from nonendemic areas, such as Los Angeles and New York, in individuals who were born in endemic areas but who had not visited those areas for several years.[23,52–54] Evidence for primary or reinfection in areas with high endemicity has been drawn from an inordinate number of cases of PDH seen with AIDS in the area.[44,51] From studies of these and other immunosuppressed individuals, such as transplant recipients, it is obvious that cure of PDH is dependent upon recovery of the cell-mediated immune deficit.[19,20] Patients with AIDS are essentially never cured of PDH, whereas patients with renal transplantation recover once immunosuppression is reversed.

As mentioned above, dissemination of yeast forms of *H capsulatum* occurs soon after infection. A primed lymphocyte macrophage system is required to keep the infection limited. In immunologically normal individuals, cell-mediated immunity may not develop. These individuals develop PDH similar to that seen in other immunosuppressed individuals. One group at particular risk of PDH consists of infants and small children.[27] This may explain the number of cases of PDH diagnosis in these individuals soon after histoplasmosis was discovered. Goodwin and colleagues have developed a spectrum of PDH based on clinical and pathologic grounds.[27] The acute, infantile form is at one extreme, with subacute in the middle and chronic PDH at the other extreme.[27] In the acute or infantile form it is rare to find granuloma formation, and the number of organisms found in reticuloendothelial tissues is high. This form corresponds to disease seen in individuals who suffer with AIDS. At the other extreme, the chronic form usually occurs in otherwise normal adults. Symptoms are prolonged and granuloma formation occurs.

Chronic pulmonary histoplasmosis has been described in patients with centrilobular emphysema.[18] This disease behaves differently from other forms of histoplasmosis. The pathogenesis of infection appears to be directly related to abnormal pulmonary architecture, which contributes to a different host response to infection. Within bullae and destroyed alveolar septa, collections of organisms occur after primary infection. These collections are poorly drained and occasionally spill into other areas of lung, causing repeated self-inoculation of the infection. Symptoms are chronic and are slow to resolve when compared to primary pulmonary histoplasmosis. Often, the areas of the lung involved correspond to those affected by tuberculosis, the apices of the upper and lower lobes.[55] Unlike primary pulmonary infection, treatment may be useful in decreasing the organism load.[56]

An excessive or exuberant chronic host response to *H capsulatum* is seen in patients with histoplasmoma, mediastinal granuloma, and mediastinal fibrosis. These forms result from inactive disease in which the host immune response is so excessive that it leads to a pathogenic disease state. Histoplasmomas are the residuals of primary pulmonary infection in which, as a result of the host response, a coin lesion is formed in the lung parenchyma. An isolated granuloma develops rings of concentric fibrosis and inflammation. Over years, this lesion calcifies, only to be inadvertently discovered on a routine chest roentgenogram. The appearance of this lesion raises the possibility of a pulmonary malignancy.[57] Previous chest roentgenograms showing the lesion years before can be helpful in the differential diagnosis. Occasionally, tomograms or CT scans that show concentric layers of calcification can be used to differentiate this lesion from pulmonary neoplasms. The lesion has a typical form of concentric calcification, the bull's eye lesion.

Excessive host response resulting in fibrosis usually occurs around the mediastinum and hilar lymph nodes, a condition called mediastinal granuloma.[58] A related condition is mediastinal fibrosis, in which there is not a lymph node nidus.[59] Due to the close proximity of vascular structures, such as the superior vena cava and the lymphatic chain, excessive fibrosis can lead to superior vena cava syndrome and obstruction of these structures. Occasionally, obstruction of a pulmonary bronchus can occur, causing atelectasis. Granulomas within the fibrous tissue have been shown to possess and slowly release *H capsulatum* antigens that are felt to stimulate this host response. As would be expected, antifungal therapy is usually of little benefit in these patients. Occasionally, symptoms become so severe that surgery is entertained only to relieve obstruction of the major vessels.

CLINICAL PRESENTATION

A listing of the various clinical conditions caused by histoplasmosis is seen in Table 2.[34] Approximately half of the patients with primary pulmonary histoplasmosis have an asymptomatic disease that can be demonstrated only retrospectively by skin testing, serology, or a compatible chest roentgenogram. The remainder have a variety of upper respiratory tract symptoms and chest roentgenographic findings that commonly occur within 10 days to 2 weeks after exposure. The clinical presentation is similar to a viral upper respiratory infection with fever, nonproductive

TABLE 2   Clinical Classification of Histoplasmosis

Pulmonary Disease	Exuberant Host Response	Progressive Disseminated Histoplasmosis
Acute	Histoplasmomas	Acute—infant type
Chronic	Mediastinal fibrosis	Subacute
	Mediastinal granuloma	Chronic—adult type

cough, myalgias, arthralgias, and headache. Depending on the degree of exposure, fever may be present. People with milder forms of primary pulmonary histoplasmosis do not usually consult physicians. The chest roentgenograms in these milder cases show focal infiltrates, sometimes nodular, and often with unilateral hilar lymphadenopathy. The white blood count shows a leukocytosis. In more severe cases, patients may appear relatively toxic with respiratory compromise and high fever. These patients usually consult a physician. It is important that the physician inquire about an exposure history 2 weeks before the symptoms began when considering the diagnosis. In more severe cases, chest roentgenograms show diffuse nodule infiltrates, and patients are hypoxic (Fig. 1). Most patients recover from primary pulmonary histoplasmosis within 1 or 2 weeks. Residua of the infection are seen in the chest roentgenogram as calcified pulmonary nodules or small calcifications in the spleen.

Erythema nodosum and erythema multiforme are skin

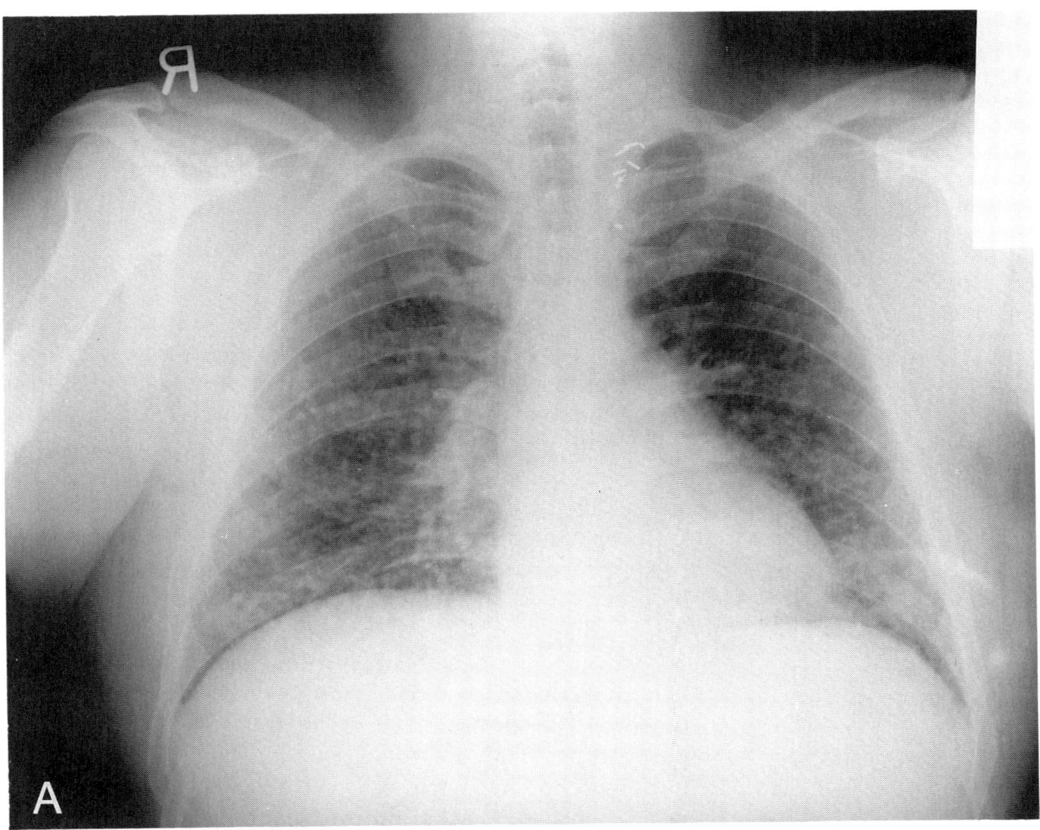

FIG. 1   Patient with acute histoplasmosis. Bilateral interstitial nodules are observed. (A) Chest roentgenogram. (*Figure continues*)

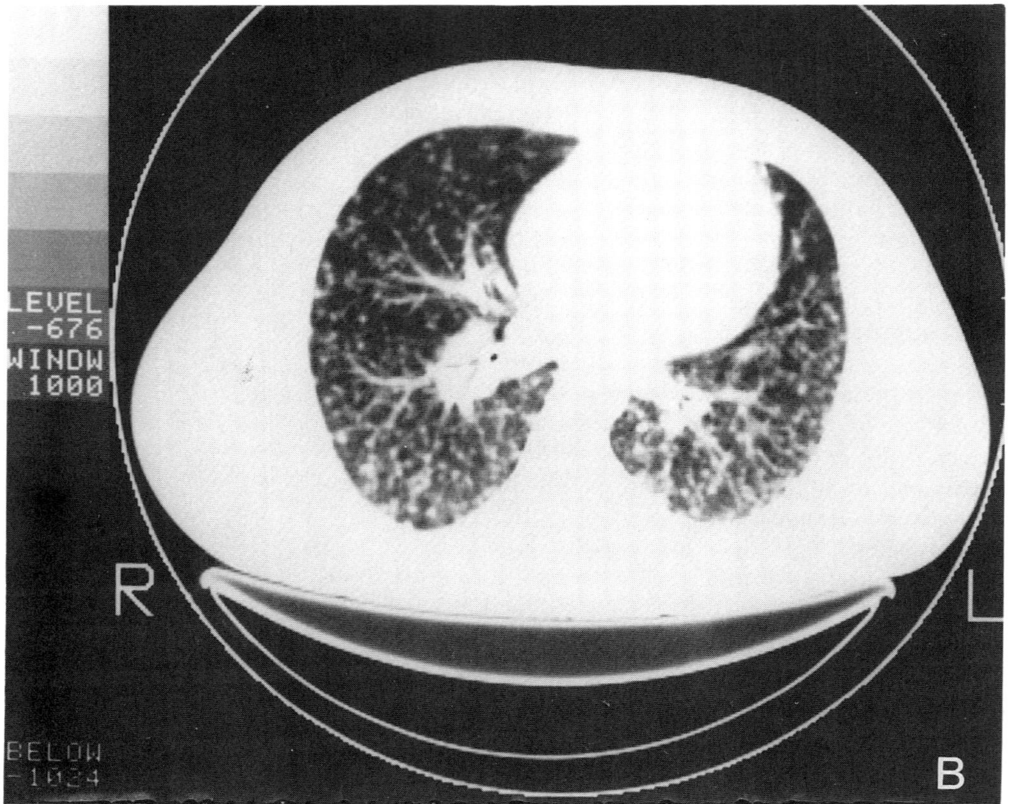

FIG. 1   (B) Computerized tomogram.

conditions that may point to outbreaks of histoplasmosis where several cases are discovered concurrently. Erythema nodosum is more commonly associated with histoplasmosis than erythema multiforme.[60] These conditions may occur with or without previous respiratory symptoms. If a chest roentgenogram is obtained, however, evidence suggestive of histoplasmosis will be seen.

In rare cases of primary pulmonary histoplasmosis, patients may develop benign pericarditis as a result of nearby involvement with hilar or periaortic lymph nodes. After a large urban outbreak of histoplasmosis in Indianapolis, Wheat and colleagues showed that up to 20% of cases of benign pericarditis in Indianapolis were due to histoplasmosis.[61] The clinical features of this disease mimic viral pericarditis. The diagnosis is suggested by mediastinal lymphadenopathy, which is not present in cases of viral pericarditis. Pericardial fluid, if sampled, is exudative and may be bloody. It is unusual to culture *H capsulatum* from pericardial fluid.[61]

Chronic pulmonary histoplasmosis usually occurs in middle-aged smokers with central lobular emphysema.[18] The initial pulmonary infection is indolent. Patients complain of sputum production, low-grade fever, and a chronic cough.[34] Weight loss and anemia may be seen. Exacerbation of pulmonary disease may occur as collections of debris from the initial infection that are trapped in cavities within the lung spill over into other noninfected areas. The chest roentgenogram reveals disease in one or more lobes of the lung.[55] The presentation, when it occurs in the upper lobes may mimic tuberculosis with cavities and air fluid levels. If left untreated, this condition may cause further respiratory compromise due to scarring. Cor pulmonale may eventually develop as a result of pulmonary hypertension.[56]

Patients with histoplasmomas usually present several years after their initial infection. Since the primary pulmonary disease is often asymptomatic, they do not recall any previous respiratory infections.[34] Diagnosis is usually made after a routine chest roentgenogram is ordered for some other reason (Fig. 2). Histoplasmomas measuring up

Histoplasmomas can grow to 1–2 cm and are usually suspected to be neoplasms. A bull's-eye calcification pattern on CT scan helps differentiate histoplasmomas from other pulmonary tumors.

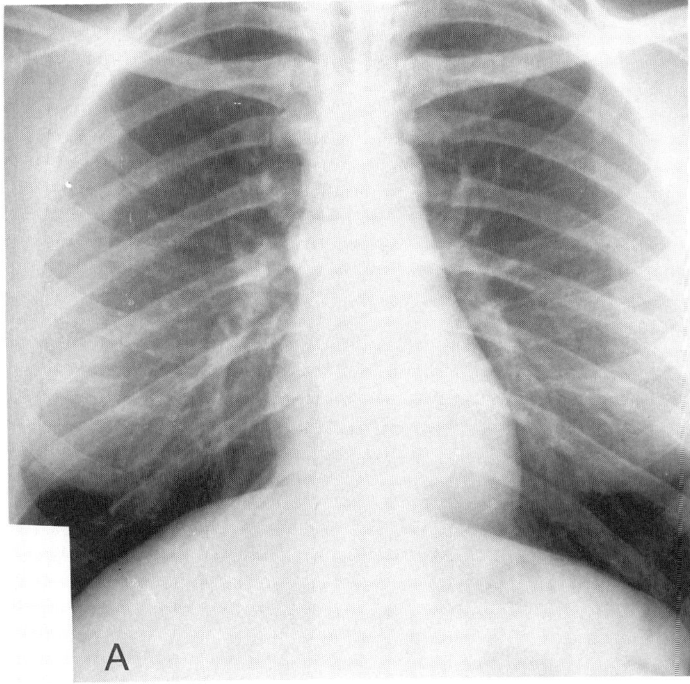

FIG. 2   Chest roentgenogram of a patient with an anterior mediastinal histoplasmoma. (A) Posteroanterior view. (*Figure continues*)

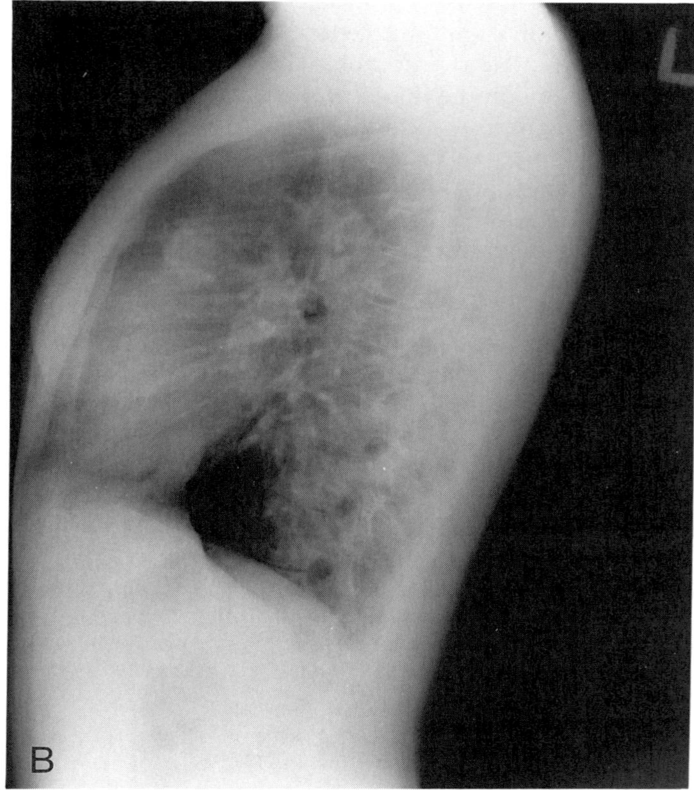

FIG. 2   (B) Lateral chest roentgenogram.

to 1 cm or 2 cm have been described.[57] In older individuals, cancer of the lung is the major condition in the differential. A careful review of previous chest roentgenograms is useful in ruling out this diagnosis. Special studies, such as CT scans and tomograms, may help differentiate a benign histoplasmoma from malignancy by the presence of a target lesion with concentric bull's-eye calcifications. Occasionally, these nodules are sampled with skinny needle biopsy or removed by thoracotomy, only to reveal granulomas with bands of calcification.

Another manifestation of excessive host response to infection is mediastinal granuloma due to histoplasmosis.[58] This condition is also usually discovered years after the original pulmonary infection. Symptoms occur if an enlarged granuloma impinges on local strictures in the mediastinum. Stricture of bronchi and pulmonary vessels may occur. The process is usually confined to the granuloma, and involvement of lung parenchyma is usually minimal.

Occasionally, surgical removal of the granuloma is necessary to improve symptoms.

Another manifestation of excessive host response is mediastinal fibrosis.[59] This is felt to be a separate disease condition from mediastinal granuloma. Again, the central structures of the mediastinum may be involved, and symptoms occur depending on the specific involvement. Symptoms of pulmonary hypertension with hemoptysis, hypoxia, and restrictive lung defects are seen with mediastinal fibrosis. Bleeding may occur from restricted arteries or veins. Occasionally, bronchi may be constricted. This may result in atelectasis. The chest roentgenogram shows a mixture of fibrosis and atelectasis (Fig. 3). Surgery for

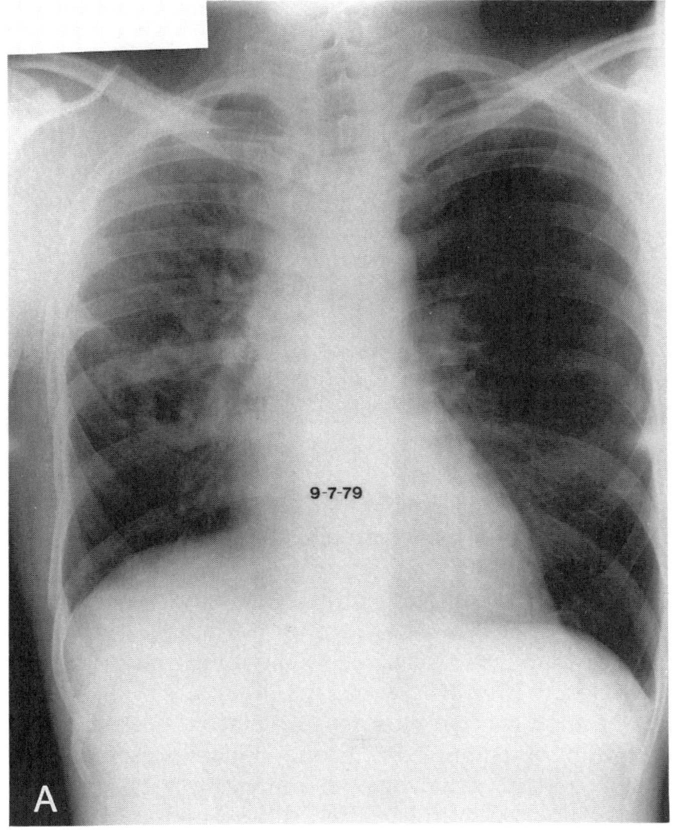

FIG. 3   Three serial chest roentgenograms of a patient with progressive mediastinal fibrosis presumed secondary to histoplasmosis. (A) Right lung fibrosis and hilar lymphadenopathy. (*Figure continues*)

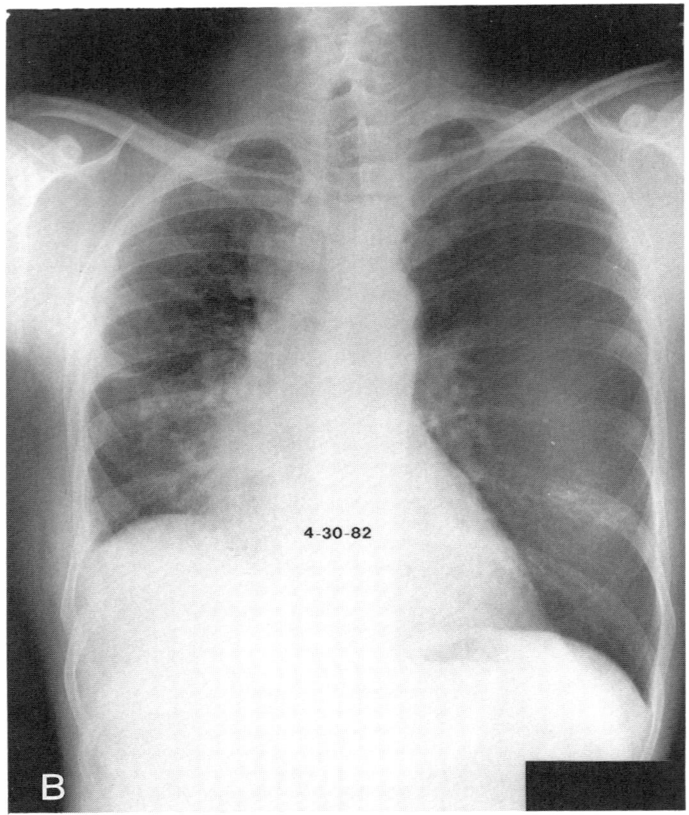

FIG. 3 (B) 2½ years later there is a progression of fibrosis, pleural reaction, and right lower-lobe atelectasis, causing shifting of the trachea to the right. (*Figure continues*)

mediastinal fibrosis is usually difficult and is not necessary as collateral vessels develop over time.

PDH occurs in two different settings. The first is immediately associated with primary pulmonary infection in which the host is unable to mount a successful cell-mediated immune response.[62] Dissemination of the organism, which occurs even with primary pulmonary disease, is left unchecked and symptoms develop that are related to multisystem involvement. The second clinical presentation occurs in a person with previous primary histoplasmosis who then becomes immunosuppressed and disseminates from sites that had previously been walled off after primary pulmonary disease.[21,63]

PDH was defined by Goodwin and coworkers prior to the AIDS epidemic.[27] They described a spectrum of disease that had clinical pathological correlates. The acute or in-

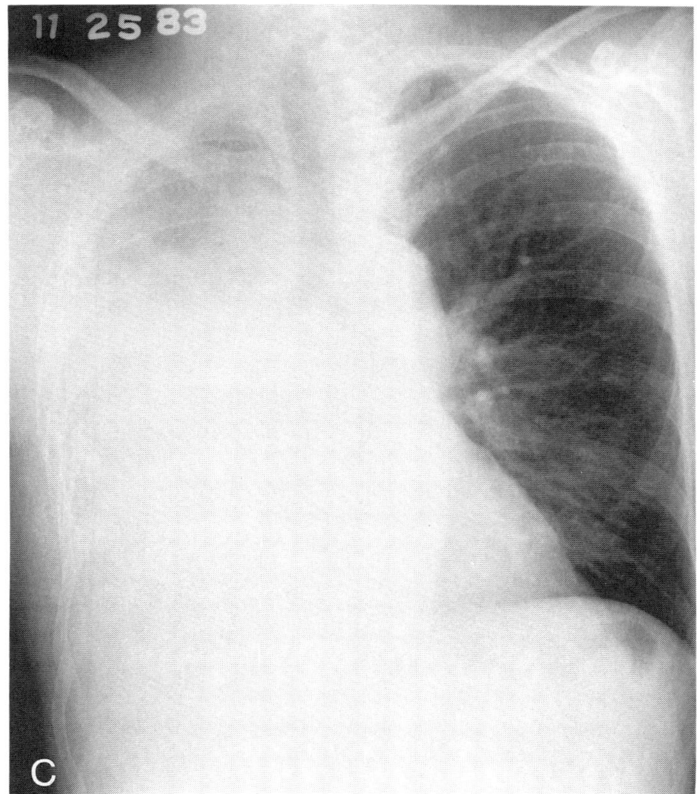

FIG. 3   (C) 1½ years later there is complete but intermittent collapse of the right middle and lower lobes. Under clinical examination, the patient had superior vena cava obstruction as well.

fantile form primarily occurred in infants and was characterized by acute onset of high fevers, malaise, and weight loss. Pulmonary symptoms occurred in approximately half of the patients. Marked enlargement of the liver and spleen was seen, and in one-third of the patients there was peripheral lymphadenopathy.[27] Laboratory manifestations of the disease included anemia, leukopenia, and thrombocytopenia, and occasionally there were abnormal liver function tests. Untreated, the course was fatal within a period of 1–2 months.

The other forms of PDH present with focal manifestations of disease, such as oral ulcerations, endocarditis, osseous lesions, and meningitis. The subacute form of PDH differs from acute PDH mainly in the degree of symptomatology.[27] There were more adults in the subacute group. Focal organ disease was seen in over half of the patients

Progressive disseminated histoplasmosis is recognized frequently in patients who are immunosuppressed as a result of chemotherapy or HIV infection.

in Goodwin's series. The physical and laboratory findings, however, were similar to those encountered in acute disease. In chronic PDH (adult type), focal organ involvement occurred in roughly 80% of the patients.[27] The most common focal presentation was oropharyngeal ulcers.[64] However, there are also cases of adrenal insufficiency, osteomyelitis, meningitis, and endocarditis. The natural course of the disease was more difficult to define than that of other forms of PDH. It was more relentless, with long periods of asymptomatic disease interrupted by manifestations of infection.

Soon after Goodwin's sentinel paper on disseminated histoplasmosis in 1980, cases of PDH were described in patients with AIDS.[23–26] The disease in persons with AIDS presented most like the acute, infantile form of PDH with acute onset of fever, malaise, and chills.[14,65] Over half of the patients have some sort of pulmonary involve-

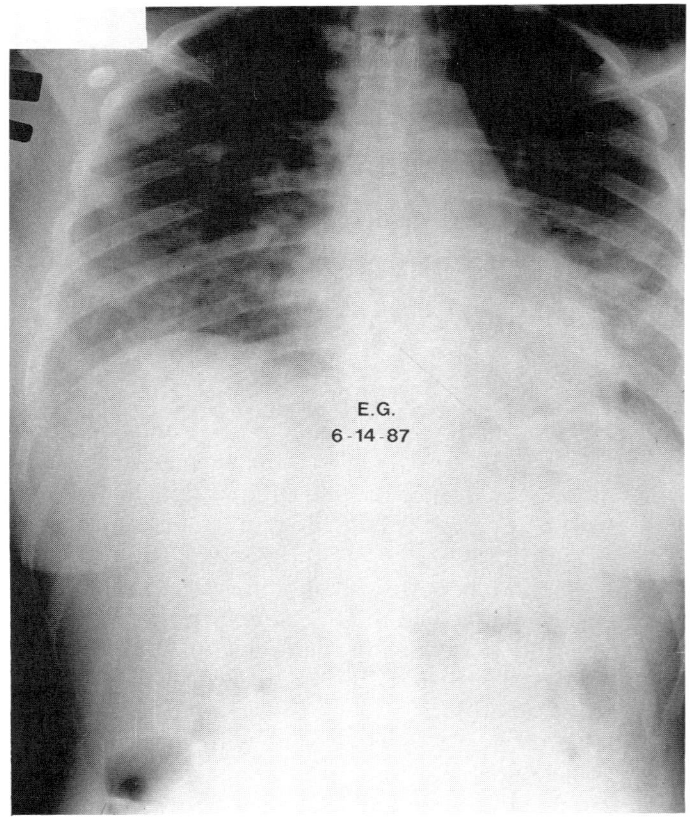

FIG. 4   Chest roentgenogram of a patient with AIDS who was found at bronchoscopy to have both *Pneumocystis carinii* pneumonia and PDH. Bilateral interstitial infiltrates are seen.

ment.[29,44,51,66] The degree of parasitization of the reticuloendothelial system in these patients is marked. Hepatosplenomegaly is found in roughly a third,[29,66] and evidence of some peripheral blood deficiency is encountered in a fourth.[29] Unlike the acute, infantile form, however, ulcerative disease is present. Skin involvement occurs in approximately 7% of patients.[29] Gastrointestinal ulcerations have been noted in around 10%, and there have been isolated descriptions of meningitis.[28,29,66] Chest roentgenograms may be normal or show diffuse reticulonodular infiltrates that may represent other pulmonary processes (Fig. 4).

There is a debate as to whether PDH in patients with AIDS occurs as primary infection or as a reactivation disease. Johnson and colleagues in Houston, an area that has low endemicity for histoplasmosis, suspect the majority of their cases presented as reactivation diseases as the result of a paucity of pulmonary presentation.[28,29] Wheat and coworkers in Indianapolis have shown serologically that a high percentage of their patients who were seen during a period of large urban outbreaks in Indianapolis may have had the disease as a result of primary infection.[44,51]

DIAGNOSIS

The diagnosis of histoplasmosis is made in three ways. First, the organism can be identified histopathologically on stains of infected tissues or cultured from the same sites. Second, evidence of disease can be obtained by a variety of serologic tests. Third, detection of histoplasma antigen from infected urine, serum, and cerebral spinal fluid is now possible using a radioimmunoassay.

The detection of *H capsulatum* in pulmonary secretions is extremely difficult. It is rare to find the organism in expectorated sputum from patients with acute pulmonary disease.[47] When positive, a 10% potassium hydroxide-(KOH) digested sputum specimen may reveal small intracellular fungi with a diameter of 2–4 μm. Culture is similarly difficult in primary pulmonary disease, and it takes between 2 and 6 weeks for the organism to grow in culture. Preliminary identification is made with the isolation of a compatible organism. Confirmatory identification requires the passage of this organism from the mycelial phase at room temperature to the yeast phase at 37°C and then back to the mycelial phase. In cases of chronic pulmonary histoplasmosis in which there are larger concentrations of organisms, identification in the sputum or by culture is more likely to be successful.

Histoplasmomas are usually diagnosed on chest roentgenogram, but confirmatory identification requires pathologic identification of the yeast from a biopsy specimen.[34,57] This may require a fine needle biopsy of a peripheral lesion under fluoroscopy or open thoracotomy. Radiologic findings that make a histoplasmoma more likely than a pulmonary neoplasm are its slow rate of growth on serial chest roentgenograms and target or bull's-eye calcifications.[34,57] Mediastinal granuloma is often diagnosed pathologically.[58] Pulmonary malignancy and lymphoma are suspected in the differential diagnosis. Mediastinal fibrosis is primarily diagnosed clinically on the basis of a compatible chest roentgenogram.[59] It is uncommon for other infectious diseases, such as tuberculosis, to cause mediastinal fibrosis.[67] The other causes of mediastinal fibrosis, including collagen vascular diseases and malignancy, need to be considered and ruled out.

In patients with PDH, the range of tissues available for sampling is much increased. Biopsies of oropharyngeal lesions and skin lesions, with or without culture, may establish the diagnosis. Lymph node biopsy, liver biopsy, and bone marrow biopsy are other very common sources of microscopic identification and culture of *H capsulatum*.[68] In patients with AIDS, the quickest diagnosis is made by skin biopsy or identification of the peripheral blood smear looking for intracellular organisms within monocytes and macrophages.[28,66] Culturing of the buffy coat utilizing the lysis centrifugation blood culture system (Dupont Isolator) is also useful.[69] Bone marrow examination is an easy and fruitful test when this diagnosis is entertained.[68] The organism can be readily found by an experienced observer utilizing specialized silver stains, such as the Gomori methenamine silver stain.

The histoplasma skin test, which was so useful as an epidemiologic tool in mapping the endemic area for histoplasmosis, is not useful for diagnosis of individual cases. A positive skin test reveals that some time in his or her life, the patient has come into contact with histoplasmosis. Additionally, a negative skin test does not rule out the diagnosis since, for primary pulmonary disease, it may take weeks after infection for skin-test reactivity to develop.[69] In patients with PDH, the histoplasma skin test is usually negative, so it is not helpful in the diagnosis.[27,62,63]

There are several serologic tests for the identification of antibody to *H capsulatum*.[71] These tests are listed in Table 3. The immunodiffusion test measures reactions to both the M and H bands. The M band is specific for a clinical picture of histoplasmosis. The H band is never found with-

TABLE 3   Diagnostic Tests for Histoplasmosis

Test	Notes
Pathologic tissue examination	Yeast forms 2–4 μm may be overlooked
Fungal culture	Initial diagnosis: 2–6 weeks, confirmation requires longer time
Histoplasmin skin test	Used for epidemiologic studies only
Immune diffusion test	M band most sensitive, not as useful as complement fixation test
Complement fixation test	Seroconversion or single titers ≥1:32 significant
Antigen detection—radioimmunoassay	Useful in patients with AIDS and PDH

AIDS, acquired immune deficiency syndrome; PDH, progressive disseminated histoplasmosis

out the M band but does add to the specificity of the diagnosis when found in conjunction with the M band. This test is not sensitive; it is positive in only 10% of proved cases, and may take 6–8 weeks to develop.[71] The complement fixation test is a better test. It measures a response to both the mycelial and yeast antigens. The yeast antigen is similar in specificity to the M band detected by the immunodiffusion test. A titer of 1:32 is highly significant. For primary pulmonary disease, the complement fixation test is the most sensitive and specific, especially if there are paired sera and a seroconversion is demonstrated.[71] For chronic pulmonary infection, the complement fixation test is invariably positive.[70] Titers are usually low and do not show a change with paired serum specimens. A negative test makes the diagnosis much less likely. The usefulness of these serologic tests in progressive disseminated infection is less clear, with less than 50% of patients with AIDS and PDH having positive serologic tests.[44,51]

Wheat and colleagues have recently developed a sensitive assay for histoplasma antigen.[72] It has been used for testing specimens from the urine, blood, and cerebral spinal fluid (CSF). The test is usually negative in patients with acute pulmonary histoplasmosis, but is very sensitive and specific for patients with PDH, especially in those with AIDS. In a recent series of PDH in patients with AIDS, histoplasma polysaccharide antigen was detected by radioimmunoassay in the urine of 67 of 69 patients (97%), blood of 39 of 46 patients (85%), and CSF of 6 of 9 patients (67%).[44,51] This assay is available only in Wheat's laboratory and can be obtained commercially by sending specimens to him.

TREATMENT

The therapy of histoplasmosis depends on an understanding of the pathogenesis of disease and the clinical course. A summary of current therapeutic recommendations for the different types of histoplasmosis is listed in Table 4. Each of these forms will be discussed in detail.

There is no effective therapy for histoplasmoma or mediastinal fibrosis.

Primary pulmonary histoplasmosis rarely requires treatment since the majority of patients are asymptomatic.[34] In those patients with mild disease, symptomatic treatment is the rule, and no antifungal therapy is necessary. In patients with severe hypoxia or high fever, AMB is the treatment of choice. Some physicians would also add corticosteroids to decrease the host's immune response.[73] Treatment with AMB should be continued for 2 or 3 weeks. A total dose of 500 mg in an adult is usually sufficient.[74] Ketoconazole, an oral triazole with activity against *H capsulatum* is ineffective in primary pulmonary disease. It is generally felt that by the time the ketoconazole has achieved efficacy, usually 2–3 weeks after starting therapy, a patient's symptoms are clinically resolved.[75]

Ketoconazole is an effective treatment for chronic pulmonary histoplasmosis. This disease is characterized by an indolent clinical course with frequent exacerbations over a period of months. The usual dose is 400 mg daily for 6 months. Ketoconazole is best given in the morning before meals as a single dose. Antacids and H_2 blockers decrease absorption. AMB is an alternative treatment. It can be given in a total dose of 2 g. The response to AMB is quicker; however, the increased toxicity of AMB precludes its use as a first-line agent except in people who are severely ill.[56]

There is no need for antifungal treatment of histoplasmoma.[57] As mentioned above, this represents old, long-

TABLE 4   Treatment of Histoplasmosis

Disease	Treatment
Acute pulmonary	Usually none required; severe cases: AMB 500 mg, total dose
Chronic pulmonary	Ketoconazole 400 mg/day for 6 months; AMB in severe cases
Histoplasmoma	None
Mediastinal granuloma	None
Mediastinal fibrosis	None; ketoconazole 400 mg/day for 6 months in rare cases
PDH	
Subacute or chronic	Ketoconazole 400 mg/day for 6 months; AMB in severe cases
Acute	AMB 1–2 g total dose
AIDS	AMB 1 g initially, then 50–80 mg/week IV for suppression
	AMB 1 g initially followed by itraconazole suppression (investigational)

AMB, amphotericin B; PDH, progressive disseminated histoplasmosis; AIDS, acquired immune deficiency syndrome

standing infection that has been walled off by the body. Likewise, there is no role for antifungal therapy in mediastinal fibrosis.[59] This condition represents the host's exuberant response to a previous infection. Corticosteroids appear to be of no benefit in preventing the continuation of the fibrotic process. There may be situations of mediastinal granuloma in which antifungal therapy with ketoconazole is of benefit.[67] One can imagine a situation in which an enlarged granuloma may be compressing a bronchus or other vital structures. Antifungal therapy may be of benefit in shrinking the infection within the lymph node and thus relieve symptoms.

The treatment of PDH depends in large part on the degree of parasitization within the individual and the level of immunosuppression. Wheat and coworkers have shown that the inability to mount a cell-mediated immune response to *H capsulatum* is a poor prognostic sign in PDH.[76] It could be expected that the patients who do the worst are those with the acute or infantile form, or patients who are severely immunocompromised, such as those with AIDS.

Ketoconazole has a role in treatment of PDH in patients that have the chronic or subacute form, or who are otherwise not severely ill.[75] A dose of 400 mg daily for 6 months is usually sufficient in these patients. Immunocompromised patients or infants with PDH should receive AMB.[27] The response to treatment with AMB is usually prompt, with the patient becoming afebrile within 2 or 3 days after starting therapy. Wheat has recently shown that patients with AIDS and PDH become afebrile after an average of 150 mg of AMB.[44,51]

In patients with AIDS and PDH, the concept of continued suppression of infection is important. As in other systemic mycoses in patients with AIDS, cryptococcosis and coccidioidomycosis, the treatment of PDH requires long-term maintenance therapy. Ketoconazole has been shown retrospectively to be ineffective as a maintenance agent.[29] Even after a total dose of 2 g of AMB, ketoconazole was unable to suppress infection and prevent relapse in these patients.[29] McKinsey has reported a prolonged clinical response in patients who received maintenance with weekly injections of 50–80 mg of AMB.[77] The major drawback to this approach is the need for an indwelling central catheter that predisposes the patient to bacterial infections.

There are several new oral agents that may prove effective in the treatment of PDH in AIDS. Itraconazole, a new imidazole, was more effective than fluconazole, another new agent, when used in a small pilot study for primary treatment.[78] In one study recently completed by

Wheat, itraconazole was effective in suppression of histoplasmosis after an initial course of AMB. This group has also advocated following patients with AIDS and PDH with histoplasma antigen determinations from the urine or blood.[44,51] An increasing titer of histoplasma antigen can be used to predict relapse in time to return to AMB therapy.

References

1. Edwards LD, Acquaviva FA, Livesay VT et al: An atlas of sensitivity to tuberculin PPD-B and histoplasmin in the United States. Am Rev Respir Dis 99(Suppl):1, 1969

2. Hammarsten JE, Hammarsten JF: Histoplasmosis recognition and treatment. Hosp Pract 26:95, 1990

3. Darling ST: A protozoan general infection producing pseudotuberculosis in the lungs and focal necrosis of the liver, spleen and lymph nodes. JAMA 46:1283, 1906

4. Darling ST: Histoplasmosis: a fatal infectious disease resembling kala azar found among natives of tropical America. Arch Intern Med 2:107, 1908

5. Darling ST: The morphology of the parasite (*Histoplasma capsulatum*) and the lesions of histoplasmosis, a fatal disease of tropical America. J Exp Med 11:515, 1909

6. Riley W, Watson CJ: Histoplasmosis of Darling, with a report of a case originating in Minnesota. Am J Trop Med Hyg 7:271, 1926

7. Dodd K, Tompkins EH: Case of histoplasmosis of Darling in an infant. Am J Trop Med Hyg 14:127, 1934

8. De Monbreun WA: The cultivation and cultural characteristics of Darling's *Histoplasma capsulatum*. Am J Trop Med Hyg 14:93, 1934

9. Parsons RJ, Zarafonetis CJD: Histoplasmosis in man. Arch Intern Med 75:1, 1945

10. Christie A, Peterson JC: Histoplasmin sensitivity. J Pediatr 29:417, 1946

11. Palmer CE: Non-tuberculous pulmonary calcification and sensitivity to histoplasmosis. Public Health Rep 60:513, 1945

12. Palmer CE: Geographic differences in sensitivity to histoplasmosis among student nurses. Public Health Rep 61:475, 1946

13. Johnson HE, Batson R: Benign pulmonary histoplasmosis. Dis Chest 14:517, 1948

14. Emmons CW: Isolation of *Histoplasma capsulatum* from soil. Public Health Rep 64:892, 1949

15. Ajello L, Zeidberg LD: Isolation of *Histoplasma capsulatum* and *Allescheria boydii* from soil. Science 113:662, 1951

16. Schwartz J, Silverman FN: The relationship of splenic calcification to histoplasmosis. N Engl J Med 252:887, 1955

17. Furcolow ML, Brasher CA: Chronic progressive (cavitary) histoplasmosis as a problem in tuberculosis sensitoriums. Am Rev Tuber Pul Dis 73:609, 1956

18. Goodwin RA Jr, Owens FT, Snell JD et al: Chronic pulmonary histoplasmosis. Medicine (Baltimore) 55:415, 1969

19. Davies SF, Khan M, Sarosi GA: Disseminated histoplasmosis in immunologically suppressed patients. Am J Med 64:923, 1978

20. Davies SF, Sarosi GA, Peterson PK et al: Disseminated histoplasmosis in renal transplant recipients. Am J Surg 137:686, 1979

21. Dismukes WE, Royal SA, Tynes BS: Disseminated histoplasmosis in corticosteroid-treated patients. JAMA 24:1495, 1979

22. Kaufman CA, Israel KS, Smith JW et al: Histoplasmosis in immunosuppressed patients. Am J Med 64:923, 1984

23. Small CB, Klein RS, Friedland GH et al: Community acquired opportunistic infections and defective cellular immunity in heterosexual drug abusers and homosexual men. Am J Med 74:433, 1983

24. Harris C, Small CB, Dlein RS: Immunodeficiency in female sexual partners of men with the acquired immunodeficiency syndrome. N Engl J Med 308:1181, 1983

25. Pasternak J, Bolivar R: Bone marrow examination and culture in the diagnosis of acquired immunodeficiency syndrome (AIDS). Arch Intern Med (letter) 143:1495, 1983

26. Kaur J, Myers AM: Homosexuality, steroid therapy and histoplasmosis. Ann Intern Med (letter) 99:567, 1983

27. Goodwin RA, Shapiro JL, Thurman GH et al: Disseminated histoplasmosis: clinical and pathologic correlations. Medicine (Baltimore) 64:923, 1978

28. Johnson PC, Khardori N, Najjar AF et al: Progressive disseminated histoplasmosis in patients with acquired immunodeficiency syndrome. Am J Med 85:152, 1988

29. Johnson PC, Hamill RJ, Sarosi GA: Clinical review: progressive disseminated histoplasmosis in the AIDS patient. Semin Respir Infect 4:139, 1989

30. Grayston JT, Furcolow ML: Occurrence of histoplasmosis in epidemics: epidemiologic studies. Am J Public Health 43:66, 1953

31. Sarosi GA, Parker JD, Tosh FE: Histoplasmosis outbreaks: their patterns. p. 123. In Balows A (ed): Histoplasmosis. Proceedings of Second National Conference. Thomas, Springfield, IL, 1971

32. Emmons CW, Klite PD, Baer GM et al: Isolation of *Histoplasma capsulatum* from bats in the United States. Am J Epidemiol 84:103, 1966

33. Disalvo AF, Bigler WB, Ajello L et al: Bat and soil studies for sources of histoplasmosis in Florida. Public Health Rep 85:1063, 1970

34. Goodwin RA Jr, Des Prez RM: Histoplasmosis: state of the art. Am Rev Respir Dis 117:929, 1978

35. Pladson TR, Stiles MA, Kuritsky JN: Pulmonary histoplasmosis: a possible risk in people who cut decayed wood. Chest 86:435, 1984

36. Gustafson TL, Kaufman L, Weeks R et al: Outbreak of acute pulmonary histoplasmosis in members of a wagon train. Am J Med 71:759, 1981

37. White FC, Hill HE: Disseminated pulmonary calcification: a report of 114 cases with observations of an antecedent pulmonary disease in 15 individuals. Am Rev Tuber Pul Dis 62:1, 1950

38. Rogers DE: The spectrum of histoplasmosis in man. Med Times 94:664, 1966

39. Hagstrom RM: Epidemiologic studies by county health departments. Miss Doctor 37:141, 1959

40. Brodsky AL, Gregg MB, Loewenstein MS et al: Outbreak of histoplasmosis associated with the 1970 Earth Day activities. Am J Med 54:333, 1973

41. Fass RJ, Saslaw SS: Earth Day histoplasmosis: a new type of urban pollution. Arch Intern Med 128:588, 1971

42. Lottenberg R, Walkman RH, Ajello L et al: Pulmonary histoplasmosis associated with exploration of a bat cave. Am J Epidemiol 110:156, 1979

43. Ward J, Weeks M, Allen D et al: Acute histoplasmosis: clinical, epidemiologic and serological findings of an outbreak associated with exposure to a fallen tree. Am J Med 66:587, 1979

44. Wheat LJ, Slama TG, Eitzen HE et al: A large urban outbreak of histoplasmosis: clinical features. Ann Intern Med 94:331, 1981

45. Tosh FE, Balhuizen J, Yates JL, Brasher CA: Primary cutaneous histoplasmosis: report of a case. Arch Intern Med 114:118, 1964

46. Tesh RB, Schneidan JD Jr: Primary cutaneous histoplasmosis. N Engl J Med 273:597, 1966

47. Reynolds RJ, Penn RL, Grafton WD, George RB: Tissue morphology of *Histoplasma capsulatum* in acute histoplasmosis. Am Rev Respir Dis 130:317, 1984

48. Baughman RP, Kim CK, Vinegar A et al: The pathogenesis of experimental pulmonary histoplasmosis to relative studies of histopathology, bronchoalveolar lavage and respiratory function. Am Rev Respir Dis 134:771, 1986

49. Schaffner A, Davis CD, Shaffner T et al: *In vitro* susceptibility of fungi to killing by neutrophil granulocytes discriminates between primary pathogenicity and opportunism. J Clin Invest 78:511, 1986

50. Gomez AK, Bullock WE, Taylor CL et al: Role of L3T4 + T cells in host defense against *Histoplasma capsulatum*. Infect Immun 56:1685, 1988

51. Wheat LJ, Connolly-Stringfield PA, Baker RL et al: Disseminated histoplasmosis in the acquired immune deficiency syndrome: clinical findings, diagnosis and treatment, and review of the literature. Medicine 69:361, 1990

52. Huang CT, McGarry T, Cooper S et al: Disseminated histoplasmosis in the acquired immunodeficiency syndrome. Report of five cases from nonendemic area. Arch Intern Med 147:1181, 1987

53. Salzman SH, Smith RL, Aranda CP: Histoplasmosis in patients with the acquired immune deficiency syndrome. Chest 93:916, 1988

54. Mandell W, Goldberg DM, Neu HC: Histoplasmosis in patients with the acquired immune deficiency syndrome. Am J Med 81:974, 1986

55. Davies SF, Sarosi GA: Acute cavitary histoplasmosis. Chest 73:103, 1978

56. Parker JD, Sarosi GA, Doto IL et al: Treatment of chronic pulmonary histoplasmosis. N Engl J Med 283:225, 1970

57. Goodwin RA Jr, Snell JD: The enlarging histoplasmoma. Am Rev Respir Dis 130:317, 1984

58. Lloyd JE, Tillman BF, Atkinson JB et al: Mediastinal fibrosis complicating histoplasmosis. Medicine (Baltimore) 67:295, 1988

59. Goodwin RA Jr, Nichell JA, Des Prez RM: Mediastinal fibrosis complicating healed primary histoplasmosis and tuberculosis. Medicine (Baltimore) 51:227, 1972

60. Sellers TF Jr, Price WN Jr, Newberry WM: An epidemic of erythema nodosum and erythema multiforme caused by histoplasmosis. Ann Intern Med 62:1244, 1965

61. Wheat LJ, Stein L, Corya BC et al: Pericarditis as a manifestation of histoplasmosis during two large urban outbreaks. Medicine (Baltimore) 62:110, 1983

62. Smith JW, Utz JP: Progressive disseminated histoplasmosis. A prospective study of 26 patients. Ann Intern Med 75:557, 1972

63. Wiseley RJ, Davey WN: Endogenous exacerbation of histoplasmosis after apparent recovery from an acute pulmonary infection. Am Rev Respir Dis 103:546, 1971

64. Reddy P, Gorelick DF, Brasher CA, Larsh H: Progressive disseminated histoplasmosis seen in adults. Am J Med 48:629, 1970

65. Johnson PC, Sarosi GA: Histoplasmosis. Semin Respir Infect 9:145, 1987

66. Nightingale SD, Parks JM, Poundersa SM et al: Disseminated histoplasmosis in patients with AIDS. South Med J 83:624, 1990

67. Davies SF: Histoplasmosis: update 1989. Semin Respir Infect 5:93, 1990

68. Davies SF, McKenna RW, Sarosi GA: Trephine biopsy of the bone marrow in disseminated histoplasmosis. Am J Med 67:617, 1979

69. Kiehn T, Wong B, Edwards FF et al: Comparative recovery of bacteria and yeast from lysis centrifugation and a conventional blood culture system. J Clin Microbiol 18:300, 1983

70. Lowell JR, Shuford EH: The value of the skin test and complement fixation test in the diagnosis of the chronic pulmonary histoplasmosis. Am Rev Respir Dis 114:1069, 1976

71. Davies SF: Serodiagnosis of histoplasmosis. Semin Respir Infect 1:9, 1986

72. Wheat LJ, Kohler RB, Tewari RP: Diagnosis of disseminated histoplasmosis by detection of *Histoplasma capsulatum* antigen in serum and urine specimens. N Engl J Med 314:83, 1986

73. George RB, Penn RL: Histoplasmosis. p. 69. In Sarosi GA, Davies SF (eds): Fungal diseases of the lung. Grune & Stratton, Orlando, 1986

74. Naylor BA: Low dose amphotericin B therapy for acute pulmonary histoplasmosis. Chest 71:404, 1977

75. National Institutes of Allergy and Infectious Diseases, Mycolosis, Study Group: Treatment of blastomycosis and histoplasmosis with ketoconazole: results of a prospective randomized clinical trial. Ann Intern Med 103:861, 1985

76. Wheat LJ, Slamma TG, Zechel ML: Histoplasmosis in the acquired immunodeficiency syndrome. Am J Med 78:203, 1987

77. McKinsey DS, Gupta MR, Riddler SA et al: Long term amphotericin B therapy for disseminated histoplasmosis in patients with the acquired immunodeficiency syndrome (AIDS). Ann Intern Med 111:655, 1989

78. Graybill JR: Histoplasmosis and AIDS. J Infect Dis 158:623, 1988

GRANULOMATOUS MENINGITIS

PATRICIA KAY SHARKEY, MD

The spectrum of etiologies capable of causing a granulomatous inflammatory response is diverse. The response can be a manifestation of infectious, allergic, autoimmune, or neoplastic disorders.[1] In many granulomatous diseases, including sarcoidosis, the underlying cause remains elusive, although the effects are clearly mediated through immunologic pathways.[1] Granulomatous inflammation is a characteristic feature of some diseases, such as sarcoidosis and tuberculosis, and is a less characteristic feature of others, such as cytomegaloviral infections. Granulomatous meningitis can be the sole manifestation of a particular disease, one manifestation of a more disseminated disease, or can represent a complication of a focal disease process spreading contiguously or rupturing into the meningeal space. Meningoencephalitis is a characteristic feature of some etiologies. The risk, presentation, course, and outcome of granulomatous meningitis is influenced by the host immunological status, the pathogen or pathogenic process, and the timing and efficacy of therapeutic intervention. In histoplasmosis, coccidioidomycosis, and tuberculosis, the degree of exposure has also been shown to affect these variables.[2–8]

In general, granuloma formation implies chronicity. The clinical presentations are usually subacute or chronic, but more acute progression can occur. By definition, a granulomatous response is an immunological reaction. Although complex, it is phylogenetically considered a primitive response, seen as a method of ingestion and removal of pathogens and persistent irritants.[1] Besides the immunologic benefits, the granulomatous response itself can result in significant morbidity and even mortality. Immunosuppressive therapy can ameliorate symptoms and signs in many of the granulomatous diseases, including some infectious causes. However, when given without concurrent specific therapy directed against the infectious pathogen, the outcome can be disastrous. Even when given concurrently with specific antiinfective agents, a price may be paid in less effective killing or clearance of the infectious pathogen. Short-term benefits clearly must be weighed

The risk, presentation, course, and outcome of granulomatous meningitis is influenced by the host immunological status, the pathogen or pathogenic process, and the timing and efficacy of therapeutic intervention.

Besides the immunologic benefits, the granulomatous response itself can result in significant morbidity and even mortality.

against long-term consequences. Nevertheless, immunosuppressives remain the mainstay of therapeutic intervention in many of the noninfectious etiologies and occasionally as adjunctive therapy in some infectious etiologies to reduce the detrimental consequences of the hosts' immunological response. However, patients with noninfectious granulomatous diseases are more susceptible to the infectious causes of granulomatous inflammation.[9,10] Immunosuppressive therapy increases a patient's susceptibility to other infections as well. Thus, immunosuppressive therapy remains the proverbial double-edged sword, with significant iatrogenic adverse consequences tempering its potential therapeutic benefits.

Various types and severities of immunosuppression or dysfunction affect granulomatous diseases in different ways.

Granulomatous inflammation is a normal immunological response to certain inciting agents. However, various types and severities of immunosuppression or dysfunction affect granulomatous diseases in different ways. Defects in the cell-mediated immune (CMI) responses, due to underlying disease or iatrogenic factors, are clearly associated with increased susceptibility to acquisition, reactivation, or dissemination of many infectious causes of granulomatous diseases. Presumably due to general depression in CMI, pregnant women are considered at increased risk of severe or disseminated coccidioidomycosis.[4] Defects in the oxidative metabolism of phagocytic cells are associated with chronic granulomatous disease, an inheritable group of disorders characterized by chronic and persistent granulomatous inflammation, with pathogens not generally associated with this type of response, including staphylococcal and gram-negative enteric organisms.[11] Delayed-type hypersensitivity (DTH) is an essential aspect of an effective immunological response to certain infectious pathogens but may be the major cause of tissue damage. Genetic factors can affect immunological responses and thus alter the risk of disease acquisition and dissemination. The higher risks of tuberculosis in patients with poor nutritional status, debilitating diseases, or at the extremes of age probably reflect their effects on the granulomatous response.[2]

The absence of a granulomatous response in patients with infection due to pathogens typically associated with this response may impart a poorer prognosis.

Patients with more severe immunosuppression are generally less capable of mounting a granulomatous inflammatory response. The absence of a granulomatous response in patients with infection due to pathogens typically associated with this response may impart a poorer prognosis due to less effective killing and clearance.[12] Such an infection, by strict definition, does not represent a granulomatous infection. Shifts in the level of immunosuppression over time can also alter the immunological response. Progressive immunological deterioration over time in patients with acquired immune deficiency syndrome (AIDS) can result in loss of an effective granulomatous response.[13,14] If acquired early in the course of immunosuppression due to AIDS, tuberculosis cases appear to be typical.[13,15] If infection occurs later in the course of AIDS, with more severe immunosuppression, tuberculosis tends to have more atypical features, including more severe pulmonary involvement, greater involvement of extrapulmonary sites including the meninges, and poorer outcomes.[13–16] Immunological recovery, following chemotherapy and remission of acute lymphocytic leukemia, has been reported in association with granulomatous histological transformation of cutaneous cryptococcoses while under antifungal treatment.[17] The distinction between granulomatous infection and infection without a granulomatous response is somewhat blurred. However, the differences in underlying pathophysiology, clinical presentation, and prognosis warrant their separation. This chapter focuses on the management of granulomatous meningitis. The principles may not be applicable to nongranulomatous presentations of a particular etiology or to other forms of chronic meningitis not involving a granulomatous inflammatory response.

A delicate balance must be achieved in host defense mechanisms to ensure a beneficial rather than a detrimental outcome. Morbidity related to granulomatous meningitis generally can be attributed to inflammatory or fibrotic host responses rather than direct tissue destruction by the pathogen. However, infectious pathogens left unchecked by these defense mechanisms result in morbidity and mortality as well. Adhesions at the base of the brain or spinal cord, a significant problem in tuberculous granulomatous meningitis, can cause constriction of nerves, obstruction of cerebrospinal fluid (CSF) flow, and infarction with a significant threat of irreparable damage. Immediate, effective treatment becomes a matter of urgency.[18]

DIAGNOSTIC ASPECTS OF GRANULOMATOUS MENINGITIS

The diagnosis of granulomatous meningitis is usually entertained in patients presenting with a chronic lymphocytic meningitis. The diagnosis is suggested by granulomas or granulomatous inflammation at other sites and is confirmed by these findings on meningeal biopsy. Due to the number of possible etiologies and persistent difficulties with diagnostic tests, determination of the specific diagnosis remains a challenge. The initial diagnostic evaluation

One of the primary concerns in the initial evaluation of granulomatous meningitis is establishing whether the patient is ill enough or progressing rapidly enough to warrant empiric treatment.

The history of underlying or prior diseases may be critical to the differential diagnosis, determination of host immunological status, and urgency of empiric therapeutic intervention.

is directed at the common and more serious etiologies. One of the primary concerns in the initial evaluation of granulomatous meningitis is establishing whether the patient is ill enough or progressing rapidly enough to warrant empiric treatment. Empiric therapy in undiagnosed cases must eventually be addressed in stable patients as well, but a period of observation may be justified. Once an etiology is discerned, subsequent management can be tailored appropriately.

The history clarifies the course, suggests the extent of involvement, identifies risk factors, and guides the remaining diagnostic evaluation. Concurrent nonmeningeal symptoms may be helpful, but neurological symptoms have limited utility in the differential diagnosis.[10] Nevertheless, neurological symptoms are helpful in suggesting the extent of disease and determining whether neurological complications, such as intracranial hypertension, cerebral vascular occlusion, hydrocephalus, or seizures, need to be addressed.[9] The history of underlying or prior diseases may be critical to the differential diagnosis, determination of host immune status, and urgency of empiric therapeutic intervention. Suspicion of a concurrent infectious granulomatous meningitis must be maintained when a possible noninfectious etiology, such as sarcoidosis, precedes the development of meningitis. The history of medications and other drug exposures, including alcohol and illicit compounds, help delineate risks. Family histories should be explored for possible genetic factors.

The exposure history is helpful in many of the infectious etiologies of granulomatous meningitis. Prior history of exposure to tuberculosis or a prior positive purified protein derivative (PPD) skin test increases the concern of this etiologic possibility and may tip the scales to early empiric therapy. The area of residence and travel history help delineate risks of endemic mycosis, such as coccidioidomycosis, histoplasmosis, blastomycosis, and paracoccidioidomycosis. Certain food ingestion may be a risk factor, such as raw or undercooked pork for cystercercosis.[9,19–23] Occupational histories may reveal exposures to particular pathogens associated with granulomatous diseases, such as meat packing and processing with brucellosis, heavy construction equipment operation, or soil exposure with sporotrichosis, histoplasmosis, and coccidioidomycosis.[3,9,24] Animal or insect exposure may be pertinent in diseases such as Lyme disease with ticks and tick-bearing animals, and toxoplasmosis with kittens and cats.[9] Exposure to multiple sexual partners may increase the risk of syphilis or AIDS and its distinctive spectrum of pathogens.

The physical examination helps to clarify the extent of

involvement and the direction and content of the remaining evaluation. Nonmeningeal sites of involvement may have a greater likelihood of yielding the etiological agent than CSF in some disseminated infections. Ophthalmologic examination may reveal evidence of choroidal tubercles, active or inactive uveitis, leukemic infiltrates, fungal exudates, or elevated intracranial pressure. Neurological examination helps to clarify the severity and extent of neurological dysfunction due to the meningitis and its complications or concurrent focal central nervous system (CNS) lesions. Findings suggestive of hydrocephalus or focal CNS lesions warrant radiographic definition before lumbar puncture. All patients should have the opening CSF pressure measured. Level of consciousness is an important prognostic index for tuberculous meningitis.[25] Nuchal rigidity directs attention to the meninges but is frequently absent. In tuberculous meningitis, it was absent in 40% of patients.[25] In patients with histoplasma meningitis, meningismus is relatively uncommon.[26]

Initial laboratory studies include routine serum chemistries and complete blood counts. Hypercalcemia, a characteristic feature of granulomatous diseases irrespective of the specific etiology, has been reported in sarcoidosis, tuberculosis, histoplasmosis, coccidioidomycosis, and disseminated candidiasis.[27–35] Adrenal insufficiency may be suggested by characteristic electrolyte abnormalities. The granulomatous infections typically involving the adrenal gland include tuberculosis, histoplasmosis, and blastomycosis.[36] Hyponatremia due to the syndrome of inappropriate antidiuretic hormone (SIADH) can occur with any meningitis but appears to be more common with tuberculous than bacterial, viral, or fungal etiologies.[37] Diabetes insipidus can occur from any of the etiologies of CNS granulomatous disease, including 10–50% of patients with neurosarcoidosis.[27] Hematological, hepatobiliary, and renal abnormalities have specific clinical implications, both diagnostic and therapeutic. Eosinophilia has been reported frequently in disseminated coccidioidomycosis but occurs in other etiologies as well.[9,10,38] Elevated angiotensin-converting enzyme (ACE) levels are characteristic of sarcoidosis occurring in the majority of patients with later stages of disease, including neurosarcoidosis. It may be a useful index in following the disease course and effectiveness of corticosteroid therapy.[27,39–41] Elevated CSF ACE levels occur in the majority of patients with neurosarcoidosis and may correlate with the clinical course and therapeutic response.[27,40,41] However, elevations in ACE levels are nonspecific and reported in many other diseases.[7,39,42]

The CSF examination should include determination of

Nonmeningeal sites of involvement may have a greater likelihood of yielding the etiological agent than CSF in some disseminated infections.

Increasing the number of samples and the volume of fluid (10–30 mL) analyzed can increase the yield of some studies, including direct examination of concentrated CSF and cultures.

cell counts and differential, glucose, and protein concentration, cytological examination, direct examination of sediment with India Ink and stains for mycobacteria and fungi, and the serologic and microbiologic studies discussed below. Increasing the number of samples and the volume of fluid (maximum, 30 mL; minimum, 10 mL) analyzed can increase the yield of some studies, including direct examination of concentrated CSF and cultures.[3,9,10,26,43,44] In one series of tuberculous meningitis, the initial specimen was positive by smear in 37% and by culture in 52% of patients, but 87% yielded acid-fast bacilli on smear when four specimens were examined.[43] A CSF pleocytosis is typically present but may be absent.[9,27,37,43–46] A lymphocytic pleocytosis is characteristic. An increased percentage of eosinophil in the CSF or even a predominance, occurs occasionally. It is characteristic of allergic etiologies and occurs occasionally in some parasitic and fungal etiologies, especially coccidioidal meningitis and cystercercosis.[9,38,47]

Hypoglycorrhachia is a characteristic finding in some etiologies and occurs occasionally or uncommonly in others.[9,10,25–27,48] It is reported in 50–95% of patients with tuberculous meningitis, in over 70% of patients with histoplasma meningitis, but in only 10–20% of those with sarcoid meningitis.[25–27] Protein elevation in the CSF is a common and nonspecific finding but occasionally may be the only abnormality initially detected.[9] Extreme elevations in CSF protein may be associated with processes like rupture of the contents of a cyst or abscess into the meningeal space or obstructive lesions.

Serological studies in patients with chronic meningitis should routinely include appropriate serum tests for lupus, syphilis, coccidioidomycosis, cryptococcosis, and histoplasmosis.

Serological studies are an important aspect of the diagnostic evaluation of granulomatous meningitis and occasionally have utility in assessing therapeutic responses or yielding prognostic information. Serological studies in patients with chronic meningitis should routinely include appropriate serum tests for lupus, syphilis, coccidioidomycosis, cryptococcoses, and histoplasmosis. Others occasionally indicated include tests for brucellosis, Lyme disease, rickettsiosis, leptospirosis, toxoplasmosis, cysticercosis, and sporotrichosis.[9,10,24,49] Serological studies performed on the CSF usually include tests for syphilis, coccidioides antibody, and cryptococcal antigen. Others may be dictated by the clinical presentation, such as tests for histoplasmosis, toxoplasmosis, cysticercosis, and sporotrichosis.[9,24] Usable serological studies for tuberculosis will likely be available within a few years.[50] Sensitivities and specificities vary among the different tests, etiologies, stages of illness, host populations, and laboratories with different levels of experience and expertise.

Twenty percent of asymptomatic patients with untreated

syphilis develop positive CSF serologies within the first 2 years, and more than 20% of these develop symptomatic neurosyphilis.[51] An array of serologic tests for syphilis include nontreponemal tests, such as antibody detection by the rapid plasma reagin (RPR) and venereal disease research laboratory (VDRL) tests and specific treponemal tests, such as the fluorescent treponemal antibody absorption (FTA-ABS) test or the microhemagglutination assay for *Treponema pallidum* (MHA-TP).[52] However, no combination of these tests can definitively establish the diagnosis of neurosyphilis.[51] The FTA-ABS is limited by its persistence in the absence of active disease and questionable utility in the CSF.[51] As with other infections in HIV-infected patients, the utility of serologic results in the diagnosis of syphilis may be limited.[53,54]

Serologic tests for Lyme disease include detection of antibodies with the indirect immunofluorescence assay (IFA) and the enzyme-linked immunosorbent assay (ELISA).[51] These tests have been poorly standardized, with reliable interpretation limited by multiple sources of variability, including the disease stage, the duration of infection, and the timing of antibiotic treatment, both within and between laboratories.[55,56] In early neurologic disease, serum IgG antibodies are almost universally present, and IgM antibodies tend to be lower and usually negative by late neurologic disease when IgG antibodies are at their highest.[51] False positive results are problematic.[51,52,55] For both leptospirosis and relapsing fever, serological studies can be helpful in confirming the diagnosis but are less useful in therapeutic decisions due to delays in seroconversion.[51] Cross-reactivity yields false positive tests for syphilis in 5–25% of patients with one of these infections.[51]

Serologic studies of brucellosis may be required to establish the diagnosis of meningitis since isolation of the organism is uncommon.[57,58] Titers are generally lower in the CSF than the serum.[57–59] The initial response is an increase in IgM by agglutination assay, the standard serological method. In chronic disease, IgG and IgA by anti-human globulin or Coombs test are often the only antibodies present.[57–59]

Efforts directed at improving the rapidity of diagnosis of tuberculous meningitis include methods permitting recognition of either mycobacterial products in clinical specimens or host responses to mycobacteria.[60,61] Procedures for detection of tuberculostearic acid in the CSF by gas chromatography/mass spectroscopy and related methods are limited by technical complexities.[61–65] Tests developed for detection of mycobacterial antigens and antibodies, including a variety of ELISA and radioimmunoassay (RIA)

Reliable interpretation of serological tests for Lyme disease have been limited by multiple sources of variability, including the disease stage, the duration of infection, and the timing of antibiotic treatment, both within and between laboratories.

techniques, offer promise in the management of tuberculous meningitis.[50,60,61,66-68] Other procedures include hemagglutination and latex agglutination immunoassay.[61,67] Adenosine deaminase is elevated in the CSF of the majority of patients with tuberculous meningitis but occasionally in other etiologies of meningitis as well.[61]

Serological studies for histoplasmosis include methods to detect antibodies and, more recently, ELISA and RIA methods for detection of histoplasma polysaccharide antigen (HPA) in body fluids.[47,69-72] Methods for antibody detection include immunodiffusion, complement-fixation (CF) tests using yeast and mycelial phase antigens, and RIAs for IgM and IgG antibodies.[47,70,72] In CNS histoplasmosis, antibodies were positive in the serum or CSF in over 60% of cases.[47] Persistence of antibody titers, despite recovery from infection and false positive and negative results in antibody tests, warrant cautious interpretation.[47] Antigen detection is a more specific and reliable index of active disease.[47,69,71] In 18 patients with CNS histoplasmosis, including 11 with meningitis, HPA was detected in the urine in 71.4%, in the blood in 37.5%, in the CSF in 40%, and by one or more of these tests in 61.1% of the cases with higher levels in the more severely immunosuppressed patients with AIDS.[47] Unfortunately, these antigen tests are not yet commercially available.

In coccidioidal meningitis, the CSF serology by CF or IDCF is positive in about 70–95% of patients, and quantitative levels can be useful in following therapeutic responses.

In all cases of suspected coccidioidomycosis, serum serology should be tested. Titers by CF greater than 1:16 suggest disseminated disease.[73,74] However, negative titers can occur with disseminated or fulminating infections, with insufficient time to mount an antibody response, or when humoral responses are compromised, such as occurs in patients with AIDS, although 80% of these patients have positive serologies.[73-76] Higher titers may correlate with a poorer prognosis.[74] Reports of cross-reactivity of the CF test with other mycotic and nonmycotic infections demonstrate the need for confirmation with immunodiffusion CF (IDCF), a more specific test.[3] In coccidioidal meningitis, the CSF serology by CF or IDCF is positive in about 70–95% of patients, and quantitative levels can be useful in following therapeutic responses.[73,74] A CF titer in the CSF at 1:2 or higher usually indicates the presence of meningitis.[3,73] Titers may vary depending on the anatomical compartment from which the CSF was obtained.[73] The tube precipitin (TP) and the immunodiffusion TP (IDTP) detect antibodies of the IgM type and are infrequently positive and of no diagnostic or prognostic value in the CSF.[3,73] The latex agglutination (LA) test yields high rates of false positive in the CSF in addition to the serum.[73] The greater sensitivity of the ELISA in detecting CSF antibodies in patients without meningitis makes it unreliable in detection of meningitis.[3,73] Methods for antigen detection are a focus of current research efforts.[3,73]

The latex cryptococcal antigen test (LCAT) is generally positive in both serum and CSF. Negative titers have been reported in cryptococcal meningitis in nonimmunosuppressed patients.[77] Higher titers correlate with poorer prognosis in non-AIDS populations, but this has not been confirmed in AIDS.[46,48,78–80] Titers may be useful in assessing therapeutic responses but may not normalize.[46,78,79] Titers greater than 1:8 after 1 month or more of therapy are associated with relapse.[78]

The slide latex agglutination (SLA) test and an enzyme immunoassay for antibody to *Sporothrix schenkii* are useful in diagnosing meningitis and following therapeutic responses.[24] Both tests were positive in the CSF in all seven patients in this series, but much higher titers were measured by enzyme immunoassay.[24] Cross activity with other pathogens appears to be minimal.[24]

Histopathology

The importance of histopathological evaluation of nonmeningeal sites of involvement in confirming the granulomatous disease and occasionally in confirming or suggesting a specific etiology deserves emphasis. Biopsies of liver, bone marrow, skin lesions, pulmonary lesions, and lymphadenopathy, when present, may demonstrate granulomas, granulomatous inflammation, caseous necrosis, or a specific organism. The finding of caseous necrosis is highly suggestive of tuberculosis but is reported with other infections such as histoplasmosis and coccidioidomycosis.[5,26] Demonstration of organisms and their morphology by special stains can improve the sensitivity and specificity of histopathology. Routinely, clinical specimens should be examined with acid-fast, hematoxylin-eosin (H and E), periodic acid-Schiff (PAS), and Gomori methenamine-silver (GMS) stains, and CSF specimens should be examined with India ink.[9,10,44] Additional histological stains for fungi are available to characterize these organisms further.

Meningeal biopsy is an aggressive diagnostic intervention for which the indications have not been clarified. It can be helpful and is warranted in some situations. In any case in which the etiology is unconfirmed and hydrocephalus requires shunting, biopsies of the meninges and accessible brain lesions should be performed at the time of the shunting procedure.[13]

The finding of caseous necrosis is highly suggestive of tuberculosis but is reported with other infections such as histoplasmosis and coccidioidomycosis.

Microbiology

The potential yield of CSF cultures varies between different pathogens, among different pathogenic processes due to the same pathogen, and between patients with differing degrees of immunological dysfunction.

The value of pursuing nonmeningeal sites of involvement in the microbiologic assessment of granulomatous meningitis also warrants emphasis. Urine cultures may be of value even in the absence of urinary tract findings in yielding mycobacteria and fungi.[9,91] Liver and bone marrow biopsies can increase the diagnostic yield in disseminated tuberculous and fungal infections.[9,10,25,26,42,81] The culture of nonmeningeal sites of involvement can confirm the specific etiology and usually have a higher yield than CSF or even meningeal biopsy culture.[9,10,25,26,42,81] The potential yield of CSF cultures varies between different pathogens, among different pathogenic processes due to the same pathogen, and between patients with differing degrees of immunological dysfunction. Microbiologic confirmation can be delayed for several weeks.

The application of monoclonal antibody techniques to early or immature cultures is an area of significant interest. In tuberculosis, histoplasmosis, and coccidioidomycosis, these techniques are already being clinically applied. Exoantigen testing of cultures in the mycelial phase may allow for earlier specific diagnosis in coccidioidomycosis.[3,73] Neucleic acid probes, applied to the recognition of mycobacteria in culture, are now available commercially.[60]

Skin Tests

Skin testing with intermediate strength PPD and coccidioidin or sperulin and controls to evaluate for anergy are routinely indicated.

Skin testing with intermediate strength PPD and coccidioidin or sperulin and controls to evaluate for anergy are routinely indicated.[9,10] Results of skin testing with PPD are less frequently positive in patients with meningitis than in patients with other sites of extrapulmonary tuberculosis.[25] The greatest utility of skin testing for delayed dermal hypersensitivity to coccidioidin or sperulin is in epidemiologic evaluations. A positive test indicates that infection has occurred but does not indicate when. Skin tests are often negative in patients with disseminated coccidioidomycosis.[3] With coccidioidomycosis and HIV infection, positive results were recorded for 6 of 36, or 17%, of patients tested.[75] Skin testing with histoplasmin antigen should be avoided because it can boost a low serological titer and it lacks diagnostic specificity.[5,7,8,70] It is more likely to be negative with greater severity of disease.[6,7,70] Skin testing with other fungal antigens has little diagnostic significance. The Kveim-Siltzbach (K-S) test, the intracutaneous injection of a previously validated saline suspension of human sarcoidal spleen or lymph node, gives rise to a nodule at the site of injection in 2–6 weeks in 40–98% of patients with active sarcoidosis.[27] The absence of mediastinal lymphadenopathy may account for a lower percentage of positive results in series of neurosarcoidosis.[27] A few false positive results have been reported in patients with regional enteritis, infectious mononucleosis, chronic lymphocytic leukemia, and nonspecific lymphadenopathy.[27]

Radiologic Studies

Radiographic studies are important in the diagnostic evaluation of granulomatous diseases. Chest radiographs are routinely indicated. Abnormalities of the pleura, lung parenchyma, and mediastinum are useful diagnostic clues and may warrant further investigation. Certain abnormalities may suggest sarcoidosis, tuberculosis, coccidioidomycosis, or histoplasmosis but generally require specific confirmation as there is considerable overlap. In tuberculous meningitis, chest radiographs are abnormal in about half of patients.[25,43] Computerized axial tomography (CT) and, more recently, magnetic resonance imaging (MRI) of the head are important diagnostic tests. These scans may reveal enhancement of basilar meninges, concurrent focal brain parenchymal lesions, or intracerebral calcification. In a series of patients with neurosarcoidosis, head CT scans were abnormal in 9 of 13, or 69%, of patients, including meningeal enhancement in four patients as well as focal parenchymal lesions, multiple low-density white-matter lesions, scattered areas of white-matter enhancement, pituitary gland enlargement, and hydrocephalus. In the same series, two of four patients had abnormalities on MRI.[27] These studies may also be useful in the diagnostic evaluation of other sites of involvement as well. Plain film radiographs and radioactive-labeled bone scans are useful in clarifying concurrent skeletal involvement.[3] Gallium radioisotope scanning abnormalities are nonspecific but are a more sensitive indicator of sarcoid activity than serum ACE levels and may suggest areas of asymptomatic extra-neurologic involvement.[27,39]

EMPIRIC THERAPY OF GRANULOMATOUS MENINGITIS

A poorer prognosis is associated with delays in therapy of tuberculous and fungal meningitis.[18,24,37,43] Empiric therapeutic trials, against the most likely treatable etiologies, are indicated when the diagnosis remains uncertain despite comprehensive evaluation or when the patient is deteriorating rapidly.[10] Sequential trials may be appropriate

Certain radiographic abnormalities may suggest sarcoidosis, tuberculosis, coccidioidomycosis, or histoplasmosis but generally require specific confirmation since there is considerable overlap.

Empiric therapeutic trials, against the most likely treatable etiologies, are indicated when the diagnosis remains uncertain despite comprehensive evaluation or when the patient is deteriorating rapidly.

in the stable patient. Interpretation of responses is difficult since they are frequently slow or incomplete even when the therapeutic choice is appropriate.[10] In most patients with chronic meningitis of undetermined etiology, an empiric trial of antituberculous therapy is warranted.[9,10] Those patients apparently responding should be treated with a full course of therapy even if all cultures remain negative. Repeat PPD after 2–4 weeks of therapy may be of value.[10] Due to its potential toxicity, some experts reserve empiric trials with amphotericin B for patients with progressive meningitis who remain undiagnosed despite meningeal biopsy.[10] However, a more liberal approach to empiric amphotericin B is frequently taken, as the role of meningeal biopsy remains unclear. The appropriate duration of therapy is difficult to determine even when the causative agent is known. At least a 10–12-week trial is probably appropriate.[10] Intrathecal administration should be considered in patients who respond to this trial but later relapse. The availability of fluconazole may tempt therapeutic trials, but fungistatic properties of this class of drugs may predispose to relapse. An empiric trial with corticosteroids is difficult to justify due to its potential catastrophic effects on unrecognized fungal meningitis.[10] Steroids should not precede trials with antituberculous therapy. Empiric treatment for seronegative syphilis has been proposed for some patients with AIDS and a compatible illness.[46]

TREATMENT ASPECTS OF GRANULOMATOUS MENINGITIS

Sarcoidosis

Spontaneous recoveries are reported with neurosarcoidosis but are unpredictable. Due to associated morbidity and mortality, treatment with steroids is generally recommended despite the lack of controlled therapeutic trials.[27] The appropriate dosage schedules and duration of treatment have not been clarified. Higher doses are generally recommended.[27] Other immunosuppressive agents and cerebral irradiation are more controversial in the treatment of neurosarcoidosis but occasionally induce remission in patients failing steroids.[27]

Tuberculosis

As with other sites, therapeutic advances have significantly improved the prognosis in tuberculous meningitis. Delays are clearly associated with poorer outcomes due to complications including adhesions, vascular occlusion, and irreversible cerebral damage.[18] Initial regimens including at least three drugs are recommended to cope with the possibility and prevent the development of resistant organisms.[18] In meningitis, drugs should be chosen that can cross and hopefully continue to cross the blood brain barrier. The recommendations of the American Thoracic Society support a two-phase therapy approach with the initial 2-month phase including isoniazid, rifampin, and pyrazinamide augmented with ethambutol when isoniazid resistance is suspected. The second phase of treatment should include isoniazid and rifampin for at least 4–7 months.[82] The adequacy of this regimen has not been substantiated by controlled therapeutic trials of meningitis. The duration of therapy must be sufficient to ensure eradication but has not been as well defined in meningitis as in other forms of the disease.[18] Favorable outcomes were reported with a 9-month regimen initially including four drugs in a series of 28 adult patients with tuberculous meningitis.[83] Longer durations are appropriate with deviations from the drug regimens suggested. The role of steroids remains controversial in the treatment of complications of tuberculous meningitis.[18,43] Steroids have clear value in reducing cerebral edema and the inflammatory exudate.[18,43] The value of steroids in reducing adhesive complications has not been established, and their use clearly can be misleading and counterproductive.[18] Surgical intervention is frequently required to deal with hydrocephalus, a common complication. A variety of other techniques have been proposed for treatment and prevention of hydrocephalus, including use of intrathecal streptokinase, streptomycin, purified protein derivative, and hyaluronidase.[84] Anecdotal reports suggest that surgical decompression of the optic chiasma constricted by basilar adhesions can be sight-preserving.[18]

Brucellosis

Doxycycline is the tetracycline of choice in treatment of brucellosis due to its good intracellular penetration and favorable pharmacokinetic properties, including suggested intrathecal secretion, but doxycycline is bacteriostatic.[57,58] Rifampin has good CSF penetration and higher intracellular levels. Synergistic effects of a rifampin-doxycycline combination have been reported. Less favorable results have been obtained with the combination of doxycycline-streptomycin-trimethoprim-sulfamethoxasole.[59] The appropriate duration of therapy has not been delineated, and relapses remain a problem. At least a 6–8-week, and typi-

Delays in treatment of tuberculous meningitis are clearly associated with poorer outcomes due to complications including adhesions, vascular occlusion, and irreversible cerebral damage.

cally longer, duration is recommended.[57–59] A suggested approach is to continue therapy until the patient recovers, CSF glucose levels normalize, CSF cell counts fall below 100/mL, and CSF antibodies begin to fall. Using this approach, the mean duration of therapy in the seven patients reported was 8.5 months, with relapses in two of six patients treated for more than 1 month.[58]

Coccidioidomycosis

Prior to the use of intrathecal amphotericin B, coccidioidal meningitis was uniformly fatal within 2 years of diagnosis.

Treatment of coccidioidomycosis is difficult. Treatment of meningeal disease is even more of a challenge. Prior to the use of intrathecal amphotericin B, coccidioidal meningitis was uniformly fatal within 2 years of diagnosis.[85] Prolonged survival can now be achieved.[3,86,87] The optimal therapy, route of administration, and dose have not been clarified. Standard therapy has included amphotericin B through intravenous and intrathecal routes. Intrathecal amphotericin B has been administered through lumbar, cisternal, and ventricular routes, the latter usually through an Ommaya reservoir.[3] Concerns regarding adequate delivery to the site of active disease, usually the basilar meninges, have been raised with the lumbar route of administration and in the setting of obstructive lesions with abnormal CSF flow patterns.[86] In addition to technical and labor requirements associated with intrathecal administration, adverse effects are expected. These include chemical meningitis, arachnoiditis, spinal cord infarction, transverse myelitis, intracisternal hemorrhage, and bacterial superinfection of mechanical access devices.[86] Concurrent intrathecal corticosteroids may ameliorate inflammatory effects, while the narcotic analgesic fentanyl can reduce headaches associated with intracisternal injections when administered concurrently by this route.[3,86,88] Doses of intrathecal amphotericin B have ranged from 0.1 mg up to 1.5 mg, with the frequency of administration ranging from three times weekly initially to once monthly for a year following conversion of CSF titers to negative.[89,90] Morbidity and mortality remain high, and relapses are common. Even with optimal treatment, the overall mortality is in the range of 30–40% and higher in the presence of hydrocephalus.[85,91]

Even with optimal treatment, the overall mortality is in the range of 30–40% and higher in the presence of hydrocephalus.

The azoles offer new alternatives in the treatment of coccidioidal meningitis. Ketoconazole, at high doses of 1,200 mg/day, has been shown to control disease in some patients unable to tolerate intrathecal administrations. However, at the higher doses apparently required, side effects are seen in more than half of the patients and can be dose-limiting.[92] Relapses have been problematic. Despite low

CSF penetration, itraconazole has been used successfully in the treatment of coccidioidal meningitis experimentally and in humans. Fluconazole, a new triazole with high CSF penetration, has also been used successfully alone and concurrently with intrathecal amphotericin B in the treatment of coccidioidal meningitis in patients with and without AIDS.[86,87,93] The optimal dose and duration and the value of adjunctive intrathecal amphotericin B have not been determined, but the reduction in potential toxicity offered by newer azoles clearly warrants further investigation. The true efficacy of any treatment cannot be determined until after years of follow-up evaluation. The value of corticosteroids has not been proven in the treatment of coccidioidal meningitis. Surgical therapy is occasionally required for management of hydrocephalus.

Histoplasmosis

It is difficult to make firm recommendations regarding the treatment of histoplasma meningitis. Conclusions from the literature are limited by the variability in reports and limited follow-up studies available in a disease in which relapses are reported up to 2 years following an initially favorable response. The literature suggests that fewer than 50% of patients treated with amphotericin B appear to be cured.[26] Of 17 cases followed for at least 1 year, in the literature reviewed by Wheat, relapse occurred in seven patients, or 41.2%.[26] Current recommendations suggest a total amphotericin B dose of at least 35 mg/kg given over 6–12 weeks.[26] There is meager evidence to support intrathecal administration.[26] Close follow-up study for at least 5 years is suggested, with repeat CSF analysis at 6 and 12 months following therapy completion.[26] Antigen studies on CSF may prove a useful tool in guiding retreatment.[26,69] Newer azoles appear promising, but clinical studies supporting efficacy in meningitis are still lacking. Years will be required before treatment regimens can be optimized to prevent relapse.

Cryptococcosis

Cryptococcal meningitis is primarily a disease of severely immunocompromised hosts; its rising incidence parallels the increase in these populations, particularly AIDS. Host factors clearly impact upon therapeutic issues. For non-AIDS patients in whom cure is the therapeutic goal, a combination regimen with amphotericin B and flucytosine is recommended. A 6-week regimen (amphotericin B at 0 3

Cryptococcal meningitis is primarily a disease of severely immunocompromised hosts; its rising incidence parallels the increases in these populations, particularly AIDS.

mg/kg/day and flucytosine at 100–150 mg/kg/day) appeared superior to a 4-week regimen.[78] Disease has been extremely difficult to cure in patients with AIDS. Lifetime suppressive therapy following an initial induction course appears to be more appropriate.[48,78,79,94–98] Due to the combined and cumulative toxicity of amphotericin B and flucytosine, oral azoles have been actively investigated in AIDS patients, contributing to the approval of fluconazole by the FDA for this indication. Itraconazole also appears promising with some studies supporting its efficacy in meningitis.[99–101] Amphotericin B lipid complex (ABLC) is just now coming into trials. It is not clear yet if an initial induction period with amphotericin B is necessary or beneficial for all patients, but some studies suggest a better outcome.[94] Although helpful, caution is warranted in the application of data obtained in trials of patients with AIDS to treatment of other populations.

References

1. Sheffield EA: The granulomatous inflammatory response. J Pathol 160:1, 1990

2. Dannenburg AM: Immune mechanisms in the pathogenesis of pulmonary tuberculosis. Rev Infect Dis 11(Suppl):S369, 1989

3. Ampel NM, Wieden MA, Galgiani JN: Coccidioidomycosis: clinical update. Rev Infect Dis 11:897, 1989

4. Wheat LJ, Slama TG, Norton JA et al: Risk factors for disseminated fatal histoplasmosis. Ann Intern Med 96:159, 1982

5. Goodwin RA, Loyd JE, Des Prez RM: Histoplasmosis in normal hosts. Medicine 60:231, 1981

6. Goodwin RA, Shapiro JL, Thurman GH et al: Disseminated histoplasmosis: clinical and pathological correlations. Medicine 59:1, 1980

7. Sathapatayavongs B, Batteiger BE, Wheat J et al: Clinical and laboratory features of disseminated histoplasmosis during two large urban outbreaks. Medicine 62:263, 1983

8. Wheat LJ, Slama TG, Eitzen HE et al: A large urban outbreak of histoplasmosis: clinical features. Ann Intern Med 94:331, 1981

9. Ellner JJ, Bennett JE: Chronic meningitis. Medicine 55:341, 1976

10. Katzman M, Ellner JJ: Chronic meningitis. p. 755. In Mandell GL, Douglas RG, Bennett JE (eds): Principles and practice of infectious diseases. 3rd ed. Churchill Livingstone Inc., New York, 1990

11. Gallin JI, Buescher ES, Seligmann BE et al: Recent advances in chronic granulomatous disease. Ann Intern Med 99:657, 1983

12. Kaufmann SHE: In vitro analysis of the cellular mechanisms involved in immunity to tuberculosis. Rev Infect Dis 11(Suppl):S448, 1989

13. Chaisson RE, Slutkin G: Tuberculosis and human immunodeficiency virus infection. J Infect Dis 159:96, 1989

14. Chaisson RE, Schecter GF, Theuer CP et al: Tuberculosis in patients with the acquired immunodeficiency syndrome. Am Rev Respir Dis 136:570, 1987

15. Theuer CP, Hopewell PC, Elias D et al: Human immunodeficiency virus infection in tuberculosis patients. J Infect Dis 162:8, 1990

16. Bishburg E, Sunderam G, Reichman LB, Kapila R: Central nervous system tuberculosis with the acquired immunodeficiency syndrome and its related complex. Ann Intern Med 105:210, 1986

17. Narisawa Y, Kojima T, Iriki A et al: Tissue changes in cryptococcoses: histologic alteration from gelatinous to suppurative granulomatous tissue response with asteroid body. Mycopathologia 106:113, 1989

18. Parsons M: The treatment of tuberculous meningitis. Tubercle 70:79, 1989

19. Sotelo J, Guerrero V, Rubio F: Neurocysticercosis: a new classification based on active and inactive forms. Arch Intern Med 145:442, 1985

20. Loo L, Braude A: Cerebral cysticercosis in San Diego, a report of 23 cases and a review of the literature. Medicine 61:341, 1982

21. Nash TE, Neva FA: Recent advances in the diagnosis and treatment of cerebral cysticercosis. N Engl J Med 311:1492, 1984

22. Brown WJ, Vogue M: Cysticercosis, a modern day plague. Pediatr Clin North Am 32:953, 1985

23. Richards FO, Schantz PM, Ruiz-Tiben E, Sorvillo FJ: Cysticercosis in Los Angeles county. JAMA 254:3444, 1985

24. Scott EN, Kaufman L, Brown AC, Muchmore HG: Serologic studies in the diagnosis and management of meningitis due to Sporothrix schenckii. N Engl J Med 317:935, 1987

25. Alvarez S, McCabe WR: Extrapulmonary tuberculosis revisited: a review of experience at Boston City and other hospitals. Medicine 63:25, 1984

26. Wheat LJ, Batteiger BE, Sathapatayavongs B: Histoplasma capsulatum infections of the central nervous system, a clinical review. Medicine 69:244, 1990

27. Chapelon C, Ziza JM, Piette JC et al: Neurosarcoidosis: signs, course, and treatment in 35 confirmed cases. Medicine 69:261, 1990

28. DeSimone DP, Brillant HL, Basile J, Bell NH: Granulomatous infiltration of the talus and abnormal vitamin D and calcium metabolism in a patient with sarcoidosis: successful treatment with hydroxychloroquine. Am J Med 87:694, 1989

29. Adams JS, Diz MM, Sharma OP: Effective reduction in the serum 1,25-dihydroxyvitamin D and calcium concentration in sarcoidosis-associated hypercalcemia with short-course chloroquine therapy. Ann Intern Med 111:437, 1989

30. Lee JC, Catanzaro A, Parthemore JG et al: Hypercalcemia in disseminated coccidioidomycosis. N Engl J Med 297:431, 1977

31. Parker MS, Dokoh F, Woolfenden JM, Buchsbaum HW: Hypercalcemia in coccidioidomycosis. Am J Med 76:341, 1984

32. Murray JJ, Heim CR: Hypercalcemia in disseminated histoplasmosis, aggravation by vitamin D. Am J Med 78:881, 1985

33. Walker JV, Baran D, Yakub YN, Freeman RB: Histoplasmosis with hypercalcemia, renal failure, and papillary necrosis: confusion with sarcoidosis. JAMA 237:1350, 1977

34. Kantarjian HM, Saad MF, Estey EH et al: Hypercalcemia in disseminated candidiasis. Am J Med 74:721, 1983

35. Abbasi AA, Chemplavil JK, Farah S: Hypercalcemia in active pulmonary tuberculosis. Ann Intern Med 90:324, 1979

36. McMurry JF, Long D, McClure R, Kotchen TA: Addison's disease with adrenal enlargement on computed tomographic scanning. Am J Med 77:365, 1984

37. Stockstill MT, Kauffman CA: Comparison of cryptococcal and tuberculous meningitis. Arch Neurol 40:81, 1983

38. Schermoly MJ, Hinthorn DR: Eosinophilia in coccidioidomycosis. Arch Intern Med 148:895, 1988

39. Sharma OP: Diagnosis of sarcoidosis. Arch Intern Med 143:1418, 1983

40. Rubinstein I, Hoffstein V: Angiotensin-converting enzyme in neurosarcoidosis. Arch Neurol 44:249, 1987

41. Oksanen V, Fyhrquist F, Somer H, Gronhagen-Riska C: Angiotensin converting enzyme in cerebrospinal fluid: a new assay. Neurology 35:1220, 1985

42. Maartens G, Wilcox PA, Benatar SR: Miliary tuberculosis: rapid diagnosis, hematologic abnormalities, and outcome in 109 treated adults. Am J Med 89:291, 1990

43. Kennedy DH, Fallon RJ: Tuberculous meningitis. JAMA 24:264, 1979

44. McGinnis MR: Detection of fungi in cerebrospinal fluid. Am J Med Suppl:129, July 28, 1983

45. Conly JM, Ronald AR: Cerebrospinal fluid as a diagnostic body fluid. Am J Med Suppl:102, 1983

46. Chuck SL, Sande MA: Infections with cryptococcus neoformans in the acquired immunodeficiency syndrome. N Engl J Med 321:794, 1989

47. Kuberski T: Eosinophil in the cerebrospinal fluid. Ann Intern Med 91:70, 1979

48. Stern JJ, Hartman BJ, Sharkey PK et al: Oral fluconazole therapy for patients with acquired immunodeficiency syndrome and cryptococcoses: experience with 22 patients. Am J Med 85:477, 1988

49. Crennan JM, Van Scoy RE: Eosinophilic meningitis caused by Rocky Mountain spotted fever. Am J Med 80:288, 1986

50. Good RC: Serologic methods for diagnosing tuberculosis (editorial). Ann Intern Med 110:97, 1989

51. Pachner AR: Spirochetal diseases of the CNS. Neurologic Clinics 4:207, 1986

52. James K: Immunoserology of infectious diseases. Clin Microbiol Rev 3:132, 1990

53. Matlow A, Rachlis AR: Syphilis serology in human immunodeficiency virus-infected patients with symptomatic neurosyphilis: case report and review. Rev Infect Dis 12:703, 1990

54. Hicks CB, Benson PM, Lupton GP, Tramont EC: Seronegative secondary syphilis in a patient infected with the human immunodeficiency virus with Kaposi sarcome: a diagnostic dilemma. Ann Intern Med 107:492, 1987

55. Magnarelli LA: Quality of Lyme disease tests (editorial). JAMA 262:3464, 1989

56. Schwartz BS, Goldstein MD, Ribeiro JMC et al: Antibody testing in Lyme disease: a comparison of results in four laboratories. JAMA 262:3431, 1989

57. Young EJ: Human brucellosis. Rev Infect Dis 5:821, 1983

58. Bouza E, Garcia de la Torre M, Parras F et al: Brucellar meningitis. Rev Infect Dis 9:810, 1987

59. Pascual J, Combarros O, Polo JM, Berciano J: Localized CNS brucellosis: report of 7 cases. Acta Neurol Scand 78:282, 1988

60. Daniel TM: Rapid diagnosis of tuberculosis: laboratory techniques applicable in developing countries. Rev Infect Dis 11(Suppl):S471, 1989

61. Daniel TM: New approaches to the rapid diagnosis of tuberculous meningitis. J Infect Dis 155:599, 1987

62. French GL, Chan CY, Cheung SW et al: Diagnosis of tuberculous meningitis by detection of tuberculostearic acid in cerebrospinal fluid. Lancet 2:117, 1987

63. French GL, Chan CY, Cheung SW, Oo KT: Diagnosis of pulmonary tuberculosis by detection of tuberculostearic acid in sputum using gas-chromatograph-mass spectrometry with selected ion monitoring. J Infect Dis 156:356, 1987

64. Elias J, De Coning JP, Vorster SA, Joubert HF: The rapid and sensitive diagnosis of tuberculous meningitis by the detection of tuberculostearic acid in cerebrospinal fluid using gas chromatograph-mass spectrometry with selective ion monitoring. Clin Biochem 22:463, 1989

65. Brooks JB, Daneshvar MI, Haberberger RL, Mikhail IA: Rapid diagnosis of tuberculous meningitis by frequency-pulsed electron-capture gas-liquid chromatography detection of carboxylic acids in cerebrospinal fluid. J Clin Microbiol 28:987, 1990

66. Wu CH, Fann MC, Lau YJ: Detection of mycobacterial antigens in cerebrospinal fluid by enzyme-linked immunosorbent assay. Tubercle 70:37, 1989

67. Chandramuki A, Bothamley GH, Brennan PJ, Ivanyi J: Levels of antibody to defined antigens of mycobacterium tuberculosis in tuberculous meningitis. J Clin Microbiol 27:821, 1989

68. Dole M, Lahiri MK, Shah MD: Enzyme-linked immunoassay for the detection of mycobacterium tuberculosis specific IgG antibody in the cerebrospinal fluid in cases of tuberculous meningitis. J Trop Pediatr 35:218, 1989

69. Wheat LJ, Kohler RB, Tweari RP et al: Significance of Histoplasma antigen in the cerebrospinal fluid of patients with meningitis. Arch Intern Med 149:302, 1989

70. Wheat J, French MLV, Kohler RB et al: The diagnostic laboratory tests for histoplasmosis. Ann Intern Med 97:680, 1982

71. Wheat LJ, Kohler RB, Tweari RP: Diagnosis of disseminated histoplasmosis by detection of histoplasma capsulatum antigen in serum and urine specimens. N Engl J Med 314:83, 1986

72. Wheat LJ, Kohler RB, French LV et al: Immunoglobulin M and G histoplasma antibody response in histoplasmosis. Am Rev Respir Dis 128:65, 1983

73. Pappagianis D, Zimmer BL: Serology of coccidioidomycosis. Clin Microbiol Rev 3:247, 1990

74. Sarosi GA, Armstrong D, Davies SF et al: Laboratory diagnosis of mycotic and specific fungal infections. Am Rev Respir Dis 132:1373, 1985

75. Roberts CJ: Coccidioidomycosis in acquired immune deficiency syndrome: depressed humeral as well as cellular immunity. Am J Med 76:734, 1984

76. Fish DG, Ampel NM, Galgiani JN et al: Coccidioidomycosis during human immunodeficiency virus infection: a review of 77 patients. Medicine 69:384, 1990

77. Berlin L, Pincus JH: Cryptococcal meningitis: false-negative antigen test results and cultures in non immunosuppressed patients. Arch Neurol 46:1312, 1989

78. Dismukes WE, Cloud G, Gallis HA et al: Treatment of cryptococcal meningitis with combination amphotericin B and flucytosine for four as compared with six weeks. N Engl J Med 317:334, 1987

79. Gupta S, Ellis M, Cesario T et al: Disseminated cryptococcal infection in a patient with hypogammaglobulinemia and normal T cell functions. Am J Med 82:129, 1987

80. Eng RHK, Bishburg E, Smith SM, Kapila R: Cryptococcal infections in patients with acquired immune deficiency syndrome. Am J Med 81:19, 1986

81. Kim JH, Langston AA, Gallis HA: Miliary tuberculosis: epidemiology, clinical manifestations, diagnosis, and outcome. Rev Infect Dis 12:583, 1990

82. Bass JB, Farer LS, Hopewell PC, Jacobs RF: Treatment of tuberculosis and tuberculosis infection in adults and children. Am Rev Respir Dis 134:355, 1986

83. Phuapradit P, Vejjajiva A: Treatment of tuberculous meningitis: role of short-course chemotherapy. Q J Med 62:249, 1987

84. Gelabert M, Castro-Gago M: Hydrocephalus and tuberculous meningitis in children. Child's Nerv Syst 4:268, 1988

85. Buss WC, Gubson TE, Gifford MA: Coccidioidomycosis of the meninges. California Medicine 72:167, 1959

86. Tucker RM, Galgiani JN, Denning DW et al: Treatment of coccidioidal meningitis with fluconazole. Rev Infect Dis 12:S380, 1990

87. Tucker RM, Denning DW, Dupont B, Stevens DA: Itraconazole therapy of chronic coccidioidal meningitis. Ann Intern Med 112:108, 1990

88. Labadie EL, Hamilon RH: Survival improvement in coccidioidal meningitis by high-dose intrathecal amphotericin B. Arch Intern Med 146:2013, 1986

89. Graybill JR, Stevens DA, Galgiani JN et al: Itraconazole treatment of coccidioidomycosis. Am J Med 89:282, 1990

90. Kelly PC: Coccidioidal meningitis. p. 163. In Stevens DA (ed): Coccidioidomycosis: a text. Plenum Medical Book Company, New York, 1980

91. Johnson RH, Brown JF, Holeman CW et al: Coccidioidal meningitis: a 25 year experience with 194 patients. p. 411. In Einstein HE, Catanzaro A (eds): Coccidioidomycosis: proceedings of the 4th international conference. The National Foundation for Infectious Diseases, Washington, DC, 1985

92. Craven PC, Graybill JR, Jorgensen JH, Dismukes WE: High-dose ketoconazole for treatment of fungal infections of the central nervous system. Ann Intern Med 98:160, 1983

93. Galgiani JN, Stevens DA, Graybill JR et al: Ketoconazole therapy of progressive coccidioidomycosis. Am J Med 84:603, 1988

94. Larsen RA, Leal MAE, Chan LS: Fluconazole compared with amphotericin B okays fucytosine for cryptococcal meningitis in AIDS. Ann Intern Med 113:183, 1990

95. Bennett JE, Dismukes WE, Duma RJ et al: A comparison of amphotericin B alone and combined with flucytosine in the treatment of cryptococcal meningitis. N Engl J Med 301:126, 1979

96. Stamm AM, Diasil RB, Dismukes WE et al: Toxicity of amphotericin B plus flucytosine in 194 patients with cryptococcal meningitis. Am J Med 83:236, 1987

97. Zuger A, Schuster M, Simberkoff MS et al: Maintenance amphotericin B for cryptococcal meningitis in the acquired immunodeficiency syndrome. Ann Intern Med 109:592, 1988

98. Sugar AM, Saunders C: Oral fluconazole as suppressive therapy of disseminated cryptococcoses in patients with acquired immunodeficiency syndrome. Am J Med 85:481, 1988

99. Denning DW, Tucker RM, Hanson LH et al: Itraconazole therapy for cryptococcal meningitis and cryptococcoses. Arch Intern Med 149:2301, 1989

100. Viviani MA, Tortorano AM, Langer M et al: Experience with itraconazole in cryptococcoses and aspergillosis. J Infect 18:151, 1989

101. Viviani MA, Tortorano AM, Giani PC et al: Itraconazole for cryptococcal infection in the acquired immunodeficiency syndrome. Ann Intern Med 106:166, 1987

PULMONARY TUBERCULOSIS

ROBERT A. ZAJAC, MD
GREGORY P. MELCHER, MD

Tuberculosis (TB) has been known as the "Captain of all men of death," and it was recognized in ancient times as an illness causing wasting, cough, fever, and hemoptysis. It is estimated that in the seventeenth and eighteenth centuries, TB may have caused one-quarter of all adult deaths in Europe.[1]

Koch was the first to describe the pathogenicity of the illness and to identify the tubercle bacillus in 1882. The antimicrobic era of TB treatment began in 1946 with the introduction of streptomycin, offering effective therapy for eradication of active disease for the first time. Isoniazid was added to the treatment regimen in 1952. The number of cases of TB decreased an average of 5% per year from 1953 to 1984. After leveling off in 1985, annual cases increased by 2.6% in 1986. Reported case rates have remained relatively stable over the past 5 years at approximately 9 cases per 100,000 population.[2] A large part of this relative increase is the result of immunosuppression induced by HIV infection,[3–6] which is discussed in another chapter. The Centers for Disease Control has recently set the goals of reducing the annual case rate to 3.5 per 100,000 population by the year 2000, and elimination of TB in the United States by the year 2010.[7]

This chapter will provide an overview of pulmonary TB. Emphasis will be placed upon recent advances in diagnosis and treatment.

Annual cases of tuberculosis increased by 2.6% in 1986, after leveling off in 1985.

EPIDEMIOLOGY

Tuberculosis is largely spread through inhalation of droplet nuclei that are infectious particles of respiratory secretions. As with any infectious disease, the determinants of infectivity relate to host factors of susceptibility, such as presence of stress, crowded living conditions, coexistent infec-

The infected individual is far more contagious in cavitary disease.

The opinions expressed herein represent those of the authors and not necessarily the U.S. Air Force or the Department of Defense.

Nonwhites are much more likely than whites to acquire new infection.

tions, malnutrition, vitamin deficiencies, presence of underlying immunosuppressive disorders, and presence or absence of natural immunity. Duration and intensity of exposure to the infected individual, lack of air circulation, and lack of environmental sunlight all increase the risk of transmission. The infected individual is far more contagious when a large burden of organisms is present, as in cavitary disease.

In the United States in 1946, with the advent of the chemotherapeutic era, which began with the introduction of streptomycin, TB was for the first time almost always a curable disease, and with treatment of index cases, transmission and secondary cases declined even further. From 1953 through 1984, the number of reported TB cases decreased by 73.6%, from 84,304 to 22,255. However, the decrease was smaller among nonwhites than whites. The risk of new infection increased in nonwhites relative to whites from 2.9 in 1953 to 5.3 in 1987.[2] The overall risk of TB for nonwhites is 4.3 times higher than that of whites or Hispanics, 4.7 times higher for American Indians and Alaskan natives, 6.4 times higher for blacks, and 11.2 times higher for Asians and pacific islanders.[2] Men are twice as likely as women to have clinical TB. Figure 1 shows the risk of TB for blacks vs whites and men vs women.

Although the increased incidence and prevalence of TB in blacks has largely been attributed to socioeconomic reasons, one recent study that addressed racial differences in

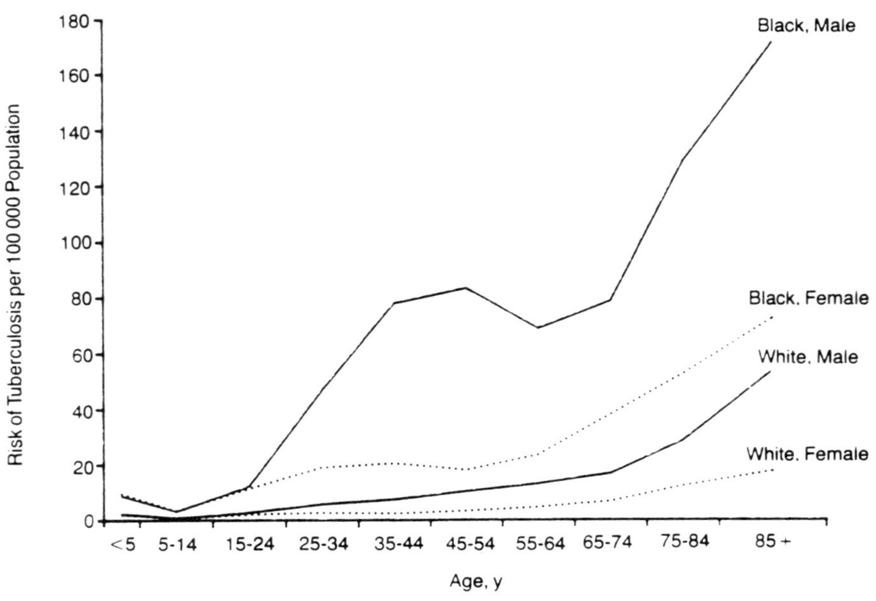

FIG. 1   The risk of tuberculosis by age and sex among blacks and whites.

susceptibility to new infection in residents of nursing homes concluded that, based on skin-test conversion in the setting of a known index case, blacks were approximately 1½ times to 1.9 times as likely to become infected.[8] The authors attempted to correct for confounding variables and found their conclusions unaltered. They cite another study showing that in vitro macrophages from blacks permit significantly more replication of *Mycobacterium tuberculosis* than whites.[9] Perhaps in TB, as in coccidioidomycosis, racial and genetic factors are important in disease susceptibility.

The greatest gains in eliminating new cases of TB have occurred in children 5–14 years of age. In adults, however, the rate of decline was progressively smaller with increasing age. In young adult age groups, risk of TB declined most among women.

In 1985, the decline in the number of reported cases was halted, and in 1986, a small increase in the number of cases of TB was reported for the first time. Since then the number of new TB cases has remained relatively stable, as shown in Figure 2.[10]

Although the exact reasons for the increase in new cases of TB are not entirely defined, it is largely attributed to an increase in the prevalence of HIV infection and AIDS (which is discussed in more detail in the chapter on TB in HIV disease) as well as the increasing prevalence of intravenous and other forms of drug abuse—most notably that of "crack" cocaine abuse.[3] In addition, increased crowding and possibly poorer nutrition and access to health care in an inner city, economically disadvantaged population may also account for part of the rise in cases. This is borne out by the fact that the annual new case rate in the United

The increase in TB cases is largely attributed to HIV/AIDS, IV drug abuse, and disadvantaged socioeconomic conditions.

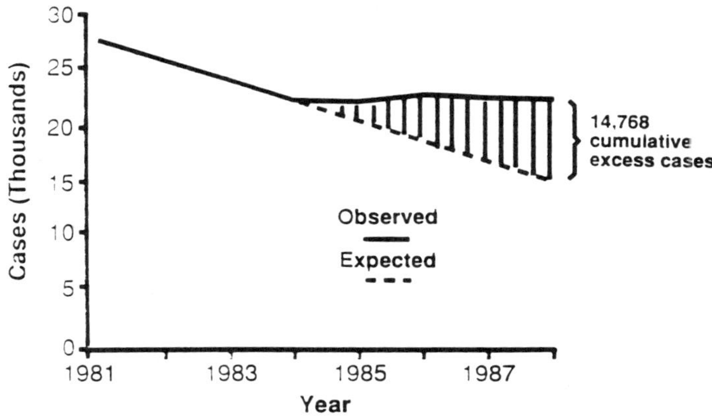

FIG. 2 Observed and expected tuberculosis cases in the United States, 1981–1988.

States in cities with over 100,000 in population was 20.7/ 100,000 vs 9.4/100,000 overall and only 6.8/100,000 in smaller cities in rural areas.[11] Other conditions that contribute to the spread of TB in the general population include an influx of immigrants from areas with high rates of TB prevalence, such as India, Southeast Asia, and Haiti, as well as the spread of disease in institutions for the mentally ill, shelters for the homeless and, to a lesser degree, nursing home facilities.[12] In at least one circumstance, it was felt that TB was transmitted in the setting of an aerosolized pentamidine treatment center for individuals with AIDS.[13]

TB remains a major health problem worldwide, accounting for an estimated 10 million new cases each year and associated with 3 million deaths, comprising 6% of all deaths.

Worldwide, TB remains a major health problem, accounting for an estimated 10 million new cases each year and associated with 3 million deaths, comprising 6% of all deaths.[14] Because of inconsistent reporting, the actual incidence and prevalence of TB is difficult to ascertain in developing countries. However, an estimate can be made using the average annual risk of TB infection (ARI). The highest ARI occurs in sub-Saharan Africa (1.5–2.5%) and Asia (1–2%). It is estimated that, with the exception of measles, more persons in developing countries die from TB each year than from other pathogens.[14]

PATHOPHYSIOLOGY

Pulmonary TB is transmitted by the inhalation of infective droplets and aerosols.

Pulmonary TB is transmitted by the inhalation of infective droplets and aerosols. Droplet nuclei are produced by infected individuals when they cough, sneeze, speak, or sing. The droplet size varies; some are in the range of 1–5 μm, allowing them to remain airborne for prolonged periods of time. Droplet nuclei of this size are able to bypass the mucosal defenses of the upper respiratory tract and the mucociliary system of the major bronchi, settling in the terminal bronchioles and alveolar spaces. Primary infection most frequently occurs in the lower lobes, the middle lobe, the lingula, and anterior segments of the upper lobes of the lung due to the relatively high airflow in these areas. Organisms initially multiply within the alveoli and pulmonary macrophages. Subsequently, the organisms migrate within macrophages via lymphatic channels to the hilar and mediastinal lymph nodes and then disseminate throughout the body. This early replicative phase occurs virtually unimpeded, as the host response is ineffective in containing the infection. Favored organs for *M tuberculosis* include bone marrow, the reticuloendothelial system, upper-lung zones, bone, brain, and the kidneys.

Subsequently, macrophages present the mycobacterial antigens to lymphocytes, which become activated. The lymphocytes proliferate and secrete lymphokines, which attract and stimulate other macrophages at the site. Activated macrophages secrete large amounts of lytic enzymes with mycobactericidal activity, and tissue necrosis results when these substances are released locally. Recruitment of activated macrophages forms tuberculous granulomas through the release of fibroblast-stimulating factors that promote collagen formation and fibrosis. The most successful cellular immune response results in the formation of Langhans giant cells, formed by fused macrophages around the tuberculous antigen. Occasionally, there is sufficient inflammatory reaction at the site of initial infection or in the hilar nodes that subsequently calcifies, resulting in the formation of the Gohn complex. More rarely, foci located in the apices or subapical sites undergo necrosis with microcalcifications called Simon foci.

Antigenic load and the vigor of the cellular immune response determine the various pathologic features of TB. Hard tubercles are formed in the setting of a small antigenic stimulus and a strong cellular response. Exudative lesions occur when the antigenic load is high, associated with a minimal host response. This may be associated with tissue necrosis resulting from the release of lytic enzymes by macrophages. The necrosis, however, is incomplete, forming a solid cheese-like mass termed caseous necrosis. The local environment within the caseous material is comprised of low oxygen tension and substances released by the cellular response; this creates a condition that is unfavorable for mycobacterial replication. If calcification occurs, replication is virtually inhibited. Although inactive in the face of cellular immunity, the organisms remain viable with the ability to renew replication if immunity wanes. However, the caseous necrotic lesions in the lung have a tendency to undergo liquefaction with resultant cavity formation, a condition that enables the organism to proliferate to very high levels (10^8–10^{11} organisms per gram of tissue). If the cavity erodes into a bronchiole, the necrotic material filled with mycobacteria can slough, resulting in bronchogenic spread to other areas of the lung. Although the apical localization of pulmonary TB is the most common residua of infection, children and the elderly may exhibit progression of the primary lower lobe process, mimicking common bacterial pneumonitis.[15]

The majority of individuals infected with *M. tuberculosis* remain asymptomatic, and the cell-mediated immune system controls further replication of the organism. Approximately 5% of infected individuals are not able to contain the infection and develop symptomatic disease within the first year after infection. Reactivation of quiescent infection

The most successful cellular immune response results in the formation of Langhans giant cells.

The various pathologic features of TB are determined by antigenic load and the vigor of the cellular immune response.

Approximately 5% of infected individuals are not able to contain the infection and develop symptomatic disease within the first year after infection.

occurs in approximately 5% at some time in their lifetime as immunity wanes, as the result of immunosuppressive therapy or another disease process associated with impaired cellular immunity. Overall, 10% of infected individuals will develop clinical disease in their lifetime.[1]

Pleural effusions may develop early in infection as a manifestation of the hypersensitivity response. Those occurring later are caused by subpleural pulmonary foci that undergo necrosis, with subsequent rupture into the pleural space. Miliary TB may occur either at the time of initial infection or later as the result of a necrotic focus eroding into a blood vessel, with resultant seeding of the bloodstream with large numbers of bacilli.

Reinfection, although not common due to the low prevalence of TB in the United States, may occur.[16] Generally, host cellular immunity is able to eradicate organisms deposited in the airways. However, depending on the intensity of the new exposure and the immune status of the host at the time of exposure, it is possible to be infected a second time.

CLINICAL AND RADIOGRAPHIC MANIFESTATIONS

Tuberculosis causes a wide range of symptoms and signs. The spectrum may range from truly asymptomatic individuals who are identified only through a history of exposure, through an abnormal chest radiograph, a positive PPD tuberculin skin test, or a positive culture, to those with an explosive pneumonic disease culminating in the adult respiratory distress syndrome (ARDS).[17] Between these two polar extremes falls a vast array of clinical presentations. Some patients have a failure-to-thrive pattern with systemic complaints, such as fatigue, anorexia, weight loss, and low-grade fevers that persist over weeks to months. Others present with an acute influenza-like illness associated with severe prostration, fevers, and chills with or without a cough. This acute pattern may be superimposed on the more chronic pattern. Occasionally, erythema nodosum or keratoconjunctivitis can be associated with the acute onset of TB. Patients may present with a more acute onset that mimics bacterial pneumonia with fevers, chills, myalgia, and purulent sputum. Others present with a fever-of-unknown-origin (FUO) pattern, which may or may not be associated with chronic cough or failure to thrive. Miliary TB secondary to hematogenous dissemination may occur with the acute onset of severe fevers, dyspnea, and cyanosis or a more chronic presentation of unexplained fever associated with distinctive hematolog-

> *Reinfection may occur, although this is uncommon due to the low prevalence of TB in the United States.*

ical abnormalities, such as pancytopenia, leukopenia, or leukemoid reaction.[17] This pattern is particularly common in elderly individuals. In pleuropulmonary TB, usually there is the gradual onset of a cough. This progresses over weeks to months and may be associated with mucoid, mucopurulent, or blood-streaked sputum. Although in the United States TB is a relatively infrequent cause of hemoptysis overall, it remains a frequent cause of massive hemoptysis. Often, patients have a dull, aching pain or tightness in the chest. Dyspnea or sharp chest pain often indicates pleural involvement with effusion.

Physical Examination

The physical examination of an individual with TB is frequently unremarkable. One may see evidence of malnutrition, stigmata of chronic obstructive pulmonary disease (COPD), alcoholism, or other serious underlying medical conditions. In the presence of pulmonary consolidation and pleural effusions, auscultation may reveal crackles, decreased breath sounds, or bronchial breath sounds. Occasionally with extensive upper-lobe cavitary disease, amphoric breath sounds can be heard over the pulmonary apices; these sounds are named for their resemblance to the sound made by blowing over the mouth of a jar.

The physical examination of an individual with TB is frequently unremarkable.

Laboratory and Pulmonary Function

The laboratory findings in TB outside of the PPD and chest radiograph are nonspecific. There is frequently a normochromic, normocytic anemia, possibly leukopenia or leukemoid reaction, and generally an elevated sedimentation rate. Hypoalbuminemia and hypergammaglobulinemia may also be present. Hyponatremia may be due to syndrome of inappropriate secretion of antidiuretic hormone (SIADH) or, much less commonly, to Addison's disease. Occasionally, hypercalcemia may be seen.[18] Pleural fluid, when tested, will often reveal an exudative effusion with elevated protein, low glucose, low pH, an elevated LDH, and a pleocytosis with lymphocytic predominance. Data regarding smear and culture sensitivity are covered in the section on Diagnosis.

There are no specific changes in pulmonary function with TB. However, in the absence of an ARDS-like pattern, one is often struck by the preservation of arterial oxygenation despite extensive lung destruction, infiltration, and cavitation, which seem to indicate a decrease in perfusion that matches the decreased ventilation to destroyed areas of the lung.[17] In the rare TB patients who present with ARDS, the pattern resembles that seen with other causes of this entity, a fact that may delay diagnosis.[19]

Chest Radiographs

Any older person who presents with chronic cough, especially with chronic pulmonary infiltrate, must be considered as possibly having TB. Unfortunately in many of these individuals, especially nursing home residents, the diagnosis of TB is not considered or detected in a timely fashion.[12,15,16] Although routine admission chest radiographs are no longer advocated in asymptomatic patients, one study showed that in a high-prevalence area for TB, in patients who presented without pulmonary symptoms but ultimately proved to have TB, the chest radiograph was abnormal and suggested the diagnosis in 90%. It is of interest that TB was not suspected initially in half of these patients, despite the abnormal chest radiograph.[20]

Examination of the chest radiograph in a patient with suspected pulmonary TB should always include an attempt to evaluate changes in chest radiograph pattern occurring over time. Therefore, the procurement and review of radiographs obtained months to years previously is invaluable. Descriptions such as "fibrotic" or "old" should be avoided when interpreting a single radiograph. However, if radiographs show no change over a period of 3–4 months to years, then these terms may be appropriately used.

Standard posteroanterior and lateral chest radiographs should be obtained. Since chronic pulmonary TB often involves apical disease, apical lordotic or oblique views may be of benefit in visualizing structures otherwise obscured by the clavicles. At times, special imaging techniques such as computerized tomography (CT) and magnetic resonance imaging (MRI) scans of the chest may be valuable for defining nodules, contours of bronchi, cavities, cysts, pleural thickening and effusion, and vascular details. Rarely, bronchography may be beneficial in definition of either bronchiectasis or bronchial stenosis. Fluoroscopy is generally limited for demonstration of diaphragmatic function or for guidance during invasive procedures.

Chest radiographs are valuable in the follow-up evaluation of response to treatment of TB; however, given the improvements in mycobacteriology and an emphasis on clinical response, they are not as important or obtained as frequently as in past decades.

The typical initial radiographic manifestation of primary pulmonary tuberculous infection is a pulmonary parenchymal infiltrate accompanied by ipsilateral mediastinal or hilar lymph node enlargement. These lymph node changes may persist longer than parenchymal infiltrates, and calcification may occur years later. Although this pattern of primary infection is typically thought of as childhood TB, recent descriptions have highlighted its frequent occurrence in immunocompromised, especially HIV-infected, individuals as well as in the elderly.[15,21]

The pattern of adult, chronic, or reactivation pulmonary TB is most commonly associated with infiltrates and cavitation in the apical-posterior segments of the upper lobes or in the superior segments of the lower lobes. In addition, nodular pulmonary infiltrates and cavitation, atelectasis,

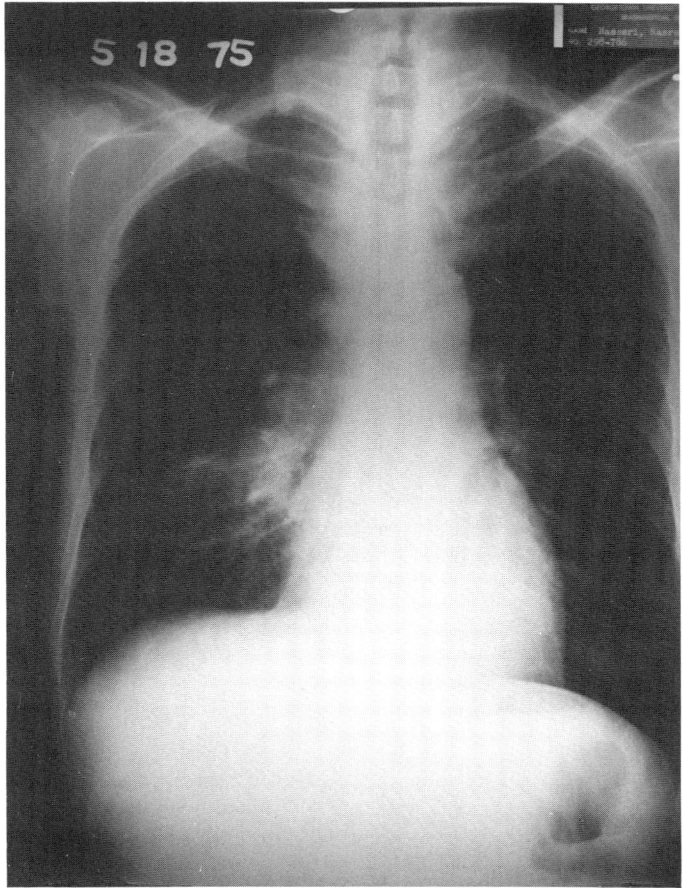

FIG. 3 Primary TB, showing right lower lobe infiltrate with ipsilateral hilar adenopathy.

Although the chest radiograph is normal in 50% of cases of miliary TB, when sequential chest radiographs are obtained over a period of several weeks in the presence of untreated disease, they generally will become abnormal.

fibrotic scarring with retraction of the hilum, and deviation of the trachea and bronchi are seen.

Miliary or hematogenous TB is characterized by diffuse, uniformly distributed, finely nodular "millet seed" densities measuring approximately 2 mm in diameter (Fig. 3). Although classically the chest radiograph is normal in 50% of cases of miliary TB, when sequential chest radiographs are obtained over a period of several weeks in the presence of untreated disease, they generally will become abnormal. Often initial changes are so subtle that the difference from normal interstitial markings is appreciated only retrospectively.

The finding in pleural disease is usually unilateral or, rarely, bilateral pleural effusion sometimes associated with pleural thickening.

Patients with pulmonary TB may present infrequently with completely normal chest radiographs. This is said to occur with greater frequency in HIV-infected individuals and rarely with endobronchial TB.

CLINICAL PATTERNS OF DISEASE

Primary Pulmonary (Childhood) Tuberculosis

Primary pulmonary TB, usually seen in childhood, typically involves the lower lobes.

As discussed above, primary pulmonary TB, most often seen in childhood, usually involves the lower lobes. Typically, there is a primary parenchymal infiltrate that, when associated with calcified regional lymph odes, is referred to as the Gohn complex. Occasionally in the recovery period, tiny calcified foci of pulmonary apical and subapical metastatic infection are seen known as Simon foci (Fig. 4).

Progressive primary pneumonia, which is seen most often in children, also occurs in immunosuppressed (such as HIV) patients and in the very elderly[22]; in normal hosts it occurs more commonly in nonwhites and in young adults. In children, one can see enlargement, occasionally massive, of the hilar and mediastinal lymph nodes, which can lead to bronchial atelectasis and distal collapse. In very young children and in infants, one can see a phenomenon known as preallergic lymphohematogenous dissemination, which causes a hyperacute miliary TB syndrome that can be complicated by tuberculous meningitis. One can also see serofibrinous pleurisy with effusion, usually unilateral, which is the result of spread of infectious and antigenic particles through lymphatics into the pleural space. Another pattern that can be seen is the seeding of the apical

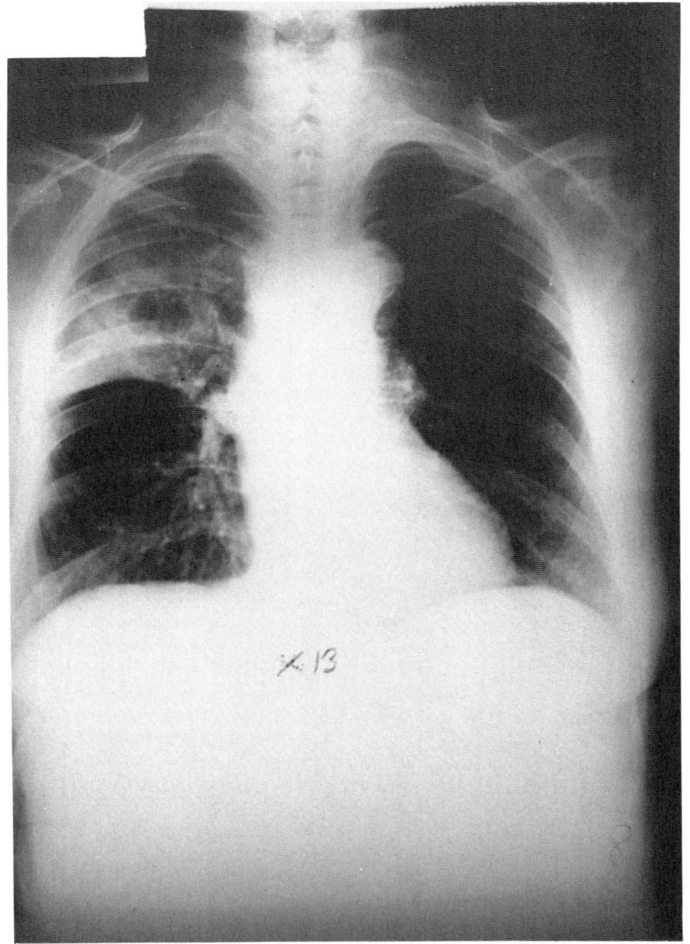

FIG. 4   Chronic upper lobe infiltrate with cavity that is characteristic of relapsing or reactivation pulmonary TB.

posterior segments of the upper lobe, leading to either latent or progressive TB, which can then evolve into the chronic or adult-type reactivation TB.

Chronic Pulmonary Tuberculosis

Chronic pulmonary TB is often localized to the apical posterior pulmonary segments. Endogenous progressive reactivation disease is felt to be the most common from areas of low TB prevalence, such as the developed countries, although exogenous reinfection with a hypersensitivity response may be important in high-prevalence countries and has recently been described in a shelter for the homeless

Chronic pulmonary TB is often localized to the apical posterior pulmonary segments.

The pivotal event in the progression of pulmonary TB is the development of a cavity.

in the United States.[16] Here one finds a patch of nodular pneumonitis that develops in the setting of a subapical collection of tubercle bacilli occurring in proximity to the clavicle or first rib. The pivotal event in the progression of pulmonary TB is the development of a cavity (Fig. 5). Within this cavity exist conditions that favor multiplication of the tubercle bacillus to levels of 10^8–10^{11} per gram of tissue, which are on the order of five or six logs higher than those found in noncavitary lesions. Cavity contents may spill into the bronchial tree and spread, causing new foci of infection to be established in the lower lobes or the

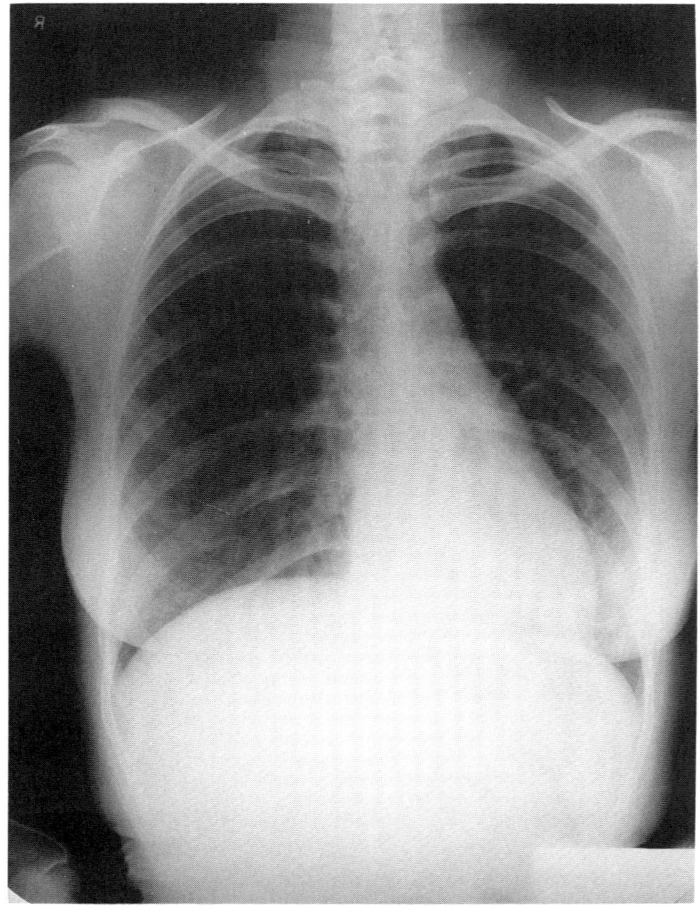

FIG. 5   Endobronchial TB with left lower lobe volume loss that can be seen as a result of bronchial obstruction from tuberculous lesion.

anterior portions of the upper lobe. However, these lesions usually have a nonprogressive course with healing and fibrosis. Spread can also occur by the lymphohematogenous route; however, this is often limited by hypersensitivity-induced thrombosis. Occasionally an established pulmonary focus can erode into a vascular channel, which is given the eponym of Rasmussen's aneurysm, causing massive hemoptysis.

At the current time, the major risk of cavities that persist after chemotherapy is comprised of superinfection with low-grade pathogens, such as aspergillus or nontuberculous mycobacteria, that can lead to hemoptysis.

Endobronchial Tuberculosis

Endobronchial TB can occur as a result of either the draining of apical cavitary disease into the lower lobes or rupture of an infected caseous lymph node into the bronchial tree. Endobronchial TB typically presents as airway obstruction or chronic cough. In its most severe form, more often seen in children, one can see bronchostenosis due to infected lymph nodes, causing distal airway collapse with consolidation. Bronchial obstruction may also be due to intrinsic stenosis from exuberant TB-induced bronchial granulation tissue (Fig. 6).

Endobronchial TB typically presents as airway obstruction or chronic cough.

On examination, one often hears localized wheezes corresponding to the segment involved. Sputum smears are usually negative, but when bronchoscopy is done, lavage may be positive up to 85% of the time. With treatment, granulation tissue and lymph nodes may regress, but scarring and stenosis, often with distal bronchiectasis may remain.

Endobronchial TB may also occur without cavitary disease or focal infiltrate as an unusual manifestation of infection in adults. When cavities occur they may have air fluid levels (uncommon in cavitary TB) due to poor drainage caused by bronchial stenosis and obstruction.[22] More often, however, endobronchial TB is associated with chest radiograph infiltrates.[23]

Sputum smears are usually negative, but when bronchoscopy is done, lavage may be positive up to 85% of the time.

Tuberculoma

Asymptomatic "coin lesions," which can be single or multiple, may develop around residual parenchymal foci of infection or as the result of fibrous encapsulation in upper-lobe caseous lesions. Rarely these lesions can continue to enlarge locally to very large- (baseball-) size masses, simulating large-cell carcinoma. Occasionally, in individuals

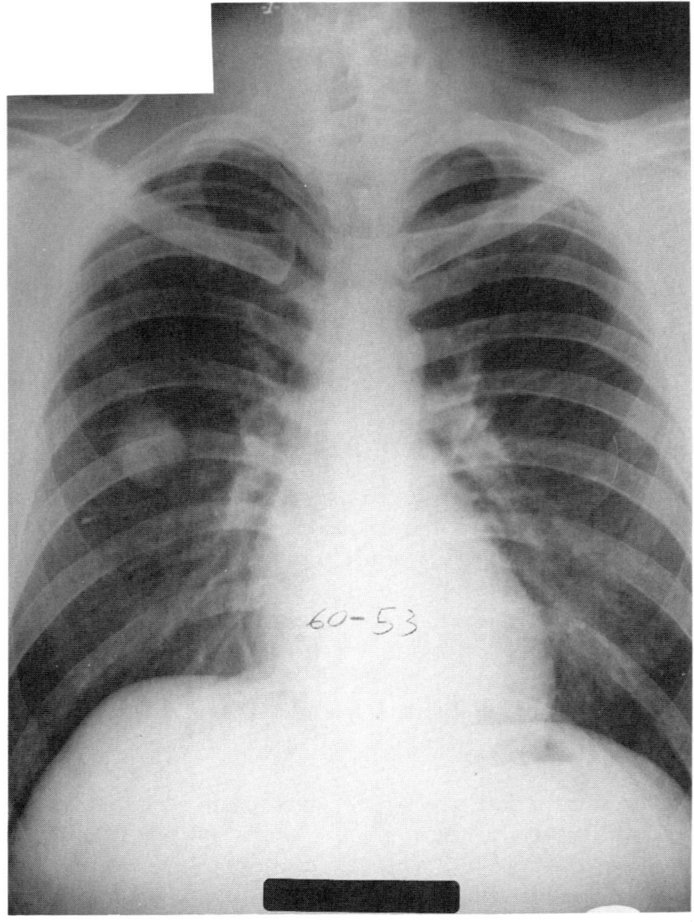

FIG. 6   Coin lesion or tuberculoma. A peripheral rounded pulmonary parenchymal density, generally asymptomatic, which may be surgically excised to exclude malignancy.

predisposed to scarring, small foci may become surrounded by concentric layers of fibrous tissue with central or concentric calcifications that resemble histoplasmosis (Fig. 7). The clinical significance of coin lesions from TB is small, with the exception of their potential for both confusion with lung carcinoma and progression to more active clinical forms.

Tuberculous Pleuritis and Empyema

Tuberculous pleuritis is one of the more common manifestations of TB. It is felt to arise when tubercule bacilli are

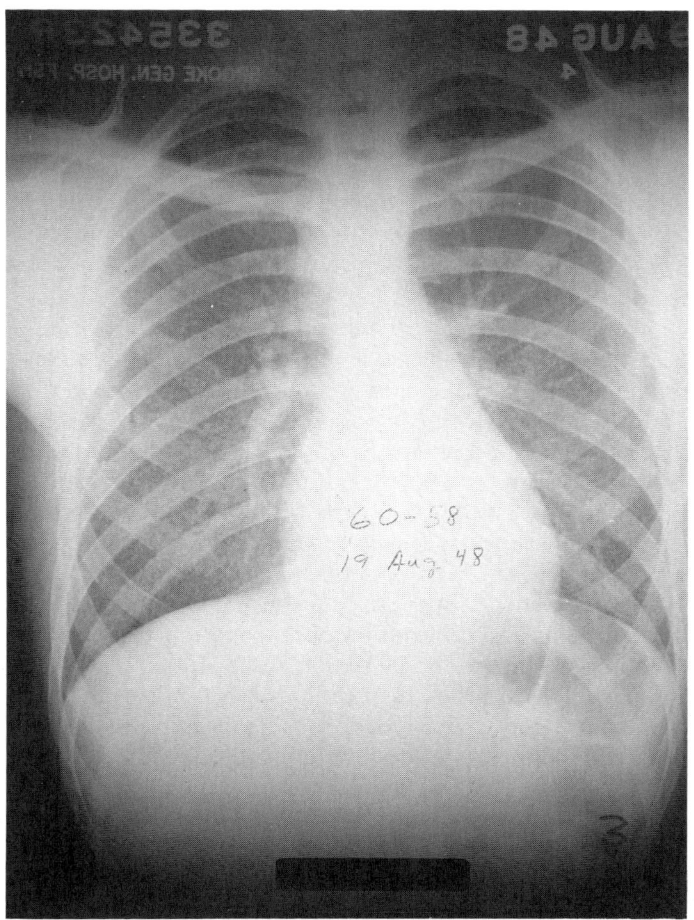

FIG. 7   Miliary or hematogenously disseminated TB typically presents as a diffuse millet-seed pattern of nodular interstitial infiltrates throughout all lung fields. Miliary TB can exist, however, in the face of a normal chest radiograph.

transported from the pulmonary parenchyma to the visceral pleura. Many times, these bacilli induce a local pleural reaction between the visceral and parietal pleura that is self-limiting, not clinically apparent, and diagnosed only at autopsy. In other patients, the presence of the bacilli and their antigens induce a more exuberant host immune response, leading to greater inflammation and more fluid accumulation. TB pleuritis is classically a disease of older children and young adults that occurs soon after the primary pulmonary infection. In approximately 10–20% of cases, one can recover AFB from bronchial secretions at the time of diagnosis.

The yield for pleural biopsy is on the order of 60–70%.

The typical clinical course is of an acute pleuritic chest pain that is sharp and severe, associated with nonproductive cough, fevers (often between 101° and 104°F), and, if the effusion is large, dyspnea. Often as the effusion increases in size, the severity of the pleuritic chest pain decreases.

Physical signs include dullness to percussion on the involved side, possible presence of a pleural friction rub with occasional findings of egophony, and rales at the upper border of the effusion.

Laboratory findings are nonspecific, although the pleural fluid generally is exudative in character, with a protein greater than 3 g/dL, and 100–1,000 white blood cells (WBCs) with a lymphocytic predominance. The yield for single pleural fluid aspirates on AFB is quite low, and the yield for culture is approximately 10–20%. The yield for pleural biopsy is higher, on the order of 60–70%. In postprimary TB pleuritis, the PPD skin test is positive in approximately 85–90% of patients.

A recent article emphasizes an alternative presentation of pleuritis as a manifestation of reactivation TB.[24] The authors noted that among 59 patients with tuberculous pleuritis, 46% had typical chest radiograph findings of reactivation TB, whereas 54% had classic postprimary TB pleuritis. Symptoms tended to be more prolonged, and pleural fluid glucose and LDH levels were more abnormal in the reactivation group; the authors felt this suggested a more chronic inflammatory process. The group with chronic pleuritis tended to have reactive PPDs less frequently (61% vs 88%) and greater evidence of granulomatous pleural inflammation with a higher bacillary burden.

The clinical course in postprimary TB pleuritis usually lasts approximately 4–12 weeks, with more rapid resolution in individuals who are treated with antituberculous medications. In chronic reactivation, TB pleuritis disease may progress to empyema.

Tuberculous Empyema

Tuberculous empyema arises as a complication of tuberculous pleurisy. Patients are occasionally asymptomatic or present with a failure-to-thrive picture. There may be a paucity of pulmonary symptoms. In contrast to simple tuberculous pleuritis, the exudate tends to be grossly purulent and contains many acid-fast bacilli. Complications include bronchopleural fistula and empyema necessitatis. Treatment is with specific antituberculous medications, chest-tube drainage, and, in severe cases in which there is pulmonary entrapment, surgical decortication.[25]

Late Complications of Treated Tuberculosis

Prior to effective chemotherapy, the major complications of pulmonary TB were recurrent disease with a prolonged wasting course, weight loss, often hemoptysis, and, in many cases, eventual death. Since the advent of effective therapy, the major complications have changed to include respiratory insufficiency, hemoptysis, and development of aspergillus mycetomas in pulmonary cavities. Generally, when respiratory insufficiency follows from TB, it accompanies disease far advanced at the time when anti-TB therapy was started, accompanies recurrent disease as the result of inadequate treatment, or stems from the extensive resection of pulmonary parenchyma. The illness, in many respects, resembles obstructive pulmonary disease with hypoxemia, later, hypercapnea, and finally, cor pulmonale with pulmonary artery hypertension. Hemoptysis is a relatively rare complication these days; however, when massive, it may necessitate emergent bronchoscopy with catheter tamponade, and definitive treatment involves surgical excision of the cavity. (See section on Surgical Treatment of TB Complications.)

Since the advent of effective therapy, the major complications of TB have included respiratory insufficiency, hemoptysis, and development of aspergillus mycetomas in pulmonary cavities.

Tuberculosis and Cancer

TB and lung cancer can often mimic each other clinically and also occur together more frequently than expected by chance. This relationship holds even after correcting for smoking habits. TB has been classically associated with scar carcinoma, although it is also associated with other histological types of lung cancer. When TB and cancer do occur together, often the diagnosis of one may obscure the other. Certain chest radiograph findings raise the possibility of cancer-complicating TB, including progression or lack of resolution of one area of disease while the remainder of lesions are regressing, the presence of a large (greater than 3-cm) mass lesion admixed with infiltrative disease, the presence of hilar nodes complicating adult chronic pulmonary TB, and the development of atelectasis.[26] When bronchoscopy is performed for the diagnosis of TB, it is important also to obtain washings and brushings for cytology. In addition, when bronchoscopy is performed for the diagnosis of suspected carcinomas, specimens should be sent for acid-fast staining and for mycobacterial culture.

DIAGNOSIS

The traditional methods for establishing the diagnosis of pulmonary TB remain: determination of exposure with the tuberculin skin test (PPD), microscopic examination of sputum smears, and culture.

New techniques applied to the field of diagnostic mycobacteriology include serological, biochemical, and molecular genetic methods.

The tuberculin skin test remains the primary method for identifying individuals infected with **M tuberculosis.**

The method used for establishing the diagnosis of pulmonary TB depends largely upon the likelihood of the presence of the disease and the duration of suspected infection. Following recent exposure, there may be a paucity of symptoms and signs, whereas the classical symptoms of fever, night sweats, weight loss associated with symptoms of cough, and possibly hemoptysis, would suggest a more advanced process. The traditional methods for establishing the diagnosis of pulmonary TB remain: determination of exposure with the tuberculin skin test (purified protein derivative, PPD), examination of sputum smears by microscopy, and culture. Recently, there have been several new techniques applied to the field of diagnostic mycobacteriology, including serological, biochemical, and molecular genetic methods, in an attempt to detect pulmonary TB. These new developments are particularly useful when a more rapid diagnosis is optimal for patient management, when the presentation of pulmonary TB is atypical, and when the standard diagnostic tests are negative; yet clinical suspicion remains high for pulmonary TB. The standard diagnostic methods for pulmonary TB will be reviewed with emphasis upon recent innovations, followed by a discussion of recent advances in diagnostic techniques.

The primary method for the identification of individuals infected with *M tuberculosis* remains the tuberculin skin test. This test relies upon the integrity of the host immune response such that upon exposure to *M tuberculosis*, T-lymphocytes are sensitized to presented antigens. This results in the characteristic subcutaneous induration of the skin when the individual is challenged by subsequent delayed hypersensitivity testing with these antigens. The product used for such testing contains cultured extracts of *M tuberculosis* and is available as old tuberculin (OT) and the PPD. OT is applied by a multiple-puncture device and is highly sensitive; this is useful for mass screening of populations at risk for TB. However, it lacks specificity; thus, a positive reaction manifested by vesiculation or the formation of papules at the site of application at 48–72 hours should always be confirmed by applying a PPD intracutaneous (Mantoux) test. Care should be exercised in applying the PPD test. A 27-gauge needle utilizing 0.1 mL of

PPD (5 TU) is injected on the volar surface of the forearm subcutaneously, creating a discrete wheal approximately 6–10 mm in diameter. The test is then interpreted 48–72 hours after application. The maximal diameter of induration in millimeters, measured transversely to the long axis of the forearm and determined by palpation, is noted and recorded. The classification of reactions to the intracutaneous Mantoux test (5 TU PPD) has recently been revised. Reactions ≥5 mm are considered positive for HIV-infected persons, recent close contacts of active TB cases, and persons with radiographic evidence of old healed TB. Reactions ≥10 mm are considered positive in persons from high prevalence areas in Asia, Africa and Latin America, intravenous drug users, indigent and medically underserved populations, high-risk racial or ethnic populations, such as blacks, Hispanics, and Native Americans, residents of long-term care facilities, and persons with underlying medical conditions placing them at increased risk for TB. These would include persons with malignancies, diabetes, mellitus, silicosis, chronic renal failure, malnutrition, gastrectomy, jejunoileal bypass, and immunosuppressive therapy. All other persons are considered positive for the test if their reaction is ≥15 mm.[17]

Several problems exist for using the PPD skin test to identify recently infected persons. There may be errors in the application of the subcutaneous antigen or in the interpretation of the induration reaction. Thus, for persons less than 35 years of age with a previous negative reaction, an increase in reaction size of 10 mm or greater in diameter within a 2-year period would be considered a PPD conversion. An increase of 15 mm or greater is required for all persons age 35 or older to be considered a conversion reaction. The booster phenomenon is a second problem in identifying newly infected persons. Delayed hypersensitivity to tuberculin may develop following exposure to any species of mycobacteria or following Calmette-Guérin bacillus (BCG) vaccination. Over years this immune response may wane, resulting in negative skin-test reactions when challenged. However, the antigenic stimulation provided by this test may recall the previously quiescent hypersensitivity so that upon subsequent testing the size of the reaction may suggest recent infection.[27] This booster effect may be seen as early as 1 week after the initial stimulating test, and the effect may last for at least a year and probably longer. Thus it is recommended that a two-step skin-testing procedure be used for adults who are to undergo periodic testing. If the reaction to the first test is negative, a second skin test should be given 7–10 days later. If this second reaction remains negative, the person is classified

The classification of reactions to the intracutaneous Mantoux test has recently been revised. Reactions ≥5 mm are considered positive for HIV-infected persons, recent close contacts of active TB cases, and persons with radiographic evidence of old healed TB.

It is recommended that a two-step skin-testing procedure be used for adults who are to undergo periodic testing.

A two-stage skin procedure should be used when testing elderly persons since the likelihood of a boosted response to the PPD skin test increases with age.

Direct staining of clinical specimens remains the most rapid and reliable method for the diagnosis of pulmonary TB.

as uninfected. A positive response with an increase of 10-mm induration from future skin testing would be interpreted as indicative of new infection over that interval of time. Since the likelihood of having a boosted response to the PPD skin test increases with age, it is suggested that a two-stage procedure be used when testing elderly persons. This may be particularly important for elderly persons at increased risk of exposure to TB, such as those who reside in nursing homes.[28,29]

Direct staining of clinical specimens remains the most rapid and reliable method for the diagnosis of pulmonary TB. This method is applicable for sputum and pleural fluid samples. The standard methodology involves a conventional acid-fast stain of clinical material, such as the Ziehl-Neelsen and Kinyoun stains. Utilization of a fluorochrome stain like the auramine-rhodamine stain increases the sensitivity of direct microscopy. Nonetheless, examination of stained specimens by microscopy is only positive in 50–80% of individuals with pulmonary TB. Despite the relatively low sensitivity of acid-fast bacteria (AFB) smears, the positive predictive value of a positive smear is nearly 100%.[30] Sometimes sputum smears are negative despite multiple samples. Gastric aspirates for AFB smear and AFB stains of urine have been advocated as useful by some, whereas others consider them unreliable due to the occurrence of false positive smears reflecting the presence of saprophytic mycobacteria. However, a recent 23-year review of gastric aspirates stained with acid-fast and fluorochrome stains for mycobacteria yielded a sensitivity of only 30% but had a specificity of 99%. Thus, a positive acid-fast stain of a gastric aspirate in the appropriate clinical setting is strongly supportive of the diagnosis of pulmonary TB.[31,32] Although mycobacteria do not stain well with common diagnostic bacterial stains, such as the Gram stain, the presence of Gram-neutral "ghosts," or faintly Gram-positive bacilli present in sputum samples stained in this manner may be suggestive of pulmonary TB.[33]

Mycobacterial cultures improve the diagnostic yield from sputum and pleural fluid specimens, with the disadvantage that confirmation of *M tuberculosis* infection may require 6–8 weeks after inoculation onto standard solid media. The radiometric culture technique, which denotes growth of mycobacteria by detecting production of $[^{14}C]$ CO_2, decreases the time required for isolation but does not differentiate *M tuberculosis* from other mycobacteria. Recently, one group has applied ELISA technology to standard radiometric culture techniques. They were able to detect antigen 5, which is contained only in *M tuberculosis* and *M bovis*, decreasing the time for specific identification to 14 days.[34] Wide application of this technique will await commercial availability of specific antiserum and antigen. Occasionally, AFB smears and cultures are negative, yet the diagnosis of TB remains highly suspected. Fiberoptic bronchoscopy with bronchoalveolar lavage for AFB smears and culture may be a useful adjunctive diagnostic technique.[35] If this technique is nondiagnostic, open lung biopsy should be considered.

It is estimated that only 50% of 8 million cases of TB annually worldwide are smear-positive.[36,37] Thus, there has been great interest in developing rapid diagnostic tests involving serological, molecular genetic, and biochemical analysis technologies. One of the major drawbacks to serological assays is the presence of cross-reacting antigens among mycobacterial species. Several groups of investigators have purified specific antigens in an attempt to improve the specificity of the assays. Utilizing an ELISA assay for serum IgM antibodies directed against the antigen A60, one group achieved a sensitivity, specificity, and positive predictive value of 76%, 98%, and 95%, respectively, for smear-negative persons clinically suspected of having TB.[38] Three groups have investigated enzyme-linked immunosorbent assays (ELISA) attempting to detect serum antibodies directed against 30–38 kD antigens of *M tuberculosis*. The first group achieved a high specificity of 96%; however the sensitivity was only 68%.[39] A second group examined the use of an ELISA for a 38-kD antigen of *M tuberculosis* in smear-negative patients. They demonstrated positive titers in 78% of patients with documented TB, and positive and negative predictive values for the assays of 90% and 91%, respectively. Further, they found that the serological results would have allowed for earlier treatment of suspected pulmonary TB and decreased the need for lung biopsy.[40] A third group of investigators assayed for IgG antibodies directed against a 30-kD native antigen and achieved a sensitivity of 70% for patients with smear-positive pulmonary TB and a specificity of 100% for control patients. However, there were two false positive tests in patients with pulmonary mycoses.[41] Determination of antibody by hemagglutination to four glycolipids and by ELISA to antigen 5 in patients with pulmonary TB is less promising, especially for smear-negative disease. The combination of these tests yields an unacceptable false positive rate of 7.9%.[42] Serodiagnosis of pulmonary TB appears promising; however, the present assays continue to be relatively insensitive for patients for whom it would be most beneficial, such as smear-negative specimens. Also, the reagents utilized in studies done thus far are not readily available for clinical use.

Serodiagnosis of pulmonary TB appears promising; however, the present assays are relatively insensitive for patients for whom it would be most beneficial, such as smear-negative specimens.

Tuberculostearic acid (TBSA) is a structural component of bacteria such as *Nocardia, Actinomyces,* and mycobacteria, and is not present in normal human tissues.[43] Because direct microscopy for TB is insensitive, investigators have been developing alternative techniques for screening specimens of patients suspected of having TB. In preliminary studies, investigators demonstrated the utility of the detection of TBSA by gas chromatography with selected ion monitoring in smear-negative, culture-positive sputum specimens. The sensitivity and specificity were 91.7% and 99.5%, respectively, for culture-positive disease, with similar results for smear-negative, culture-positive patients.[44] This group recently compared the assay to standard fluorochrome stains of bronchial washings and bronchoalveolar lavage specimens for the rapid diagnosis of pulmonary TB. The sensitivity of the assay for any one specimen remained low; however, when both were combined, the sensitivity was 96%, with a specificity and positive predictive value of 100%.[45] The TBSA assay was subsequently applied to the examination of sputum, pleural fluid, and bronchial washings. They detected TBSA in 90% of sputum samples, 75% of pleural fluid samples, and 68% of bronchial washings from patients with active pulmonary TB. For smear-negative, culture-negative samples, the assay was positive in 71% of cases.[46] Thus, this technique appears to be promising as a rapid diagnostic test for TB. Two drawbacks to the methodology are the expensive and technologically complex equipment required to perform the assay, and that the assay does not differentiate between the various species of mycobacteria.

The differentiation of tuberculous pleural effusion from malignant and benign effusions is often difficult. An attempt has been made to differentiate these entities by biochemical assays. Adenosine deaminase is an enzyme essential for the conversion of adenosine to inosine, which, in turn, is necessary for lymphocyte differentiation and proliferation. The measurement of pleural fluid adenosine deaminase activity (ADA) is a reflection of lymphocyte activation locally. Lysozyme is an enzyme with bacteriolytic properties and reflects the activity of fresh granulomas. The determination of pleural ADA[47,48] and pleural lysozyme, combined with the pleural/serum lysozyme ratio (Lp/Ls)[49–52] have been purported to be useful in differentiating tuberculous from nontuberculous effusions. Recently, the combination of these assays was measured simultaneously in 138 patients with pleural effusions, of which 61 were tuberculous. Through simultaneous determination of both parameters, they were successful in separating tuberculous effusions from those caused by other processes in most instances. Although empyema had over-lapping values of Lp/Ls, they were easily differentiated by cell count and Gram stain. Several adenocarcinomas also had elevated levels of ADA or Lp/Ls, but not both simultaneously. Further, there was good correlation between the two tests for tuberculous pleuritis.[53]

DNA amplification by polymerase chain reaction (PCR) of specific genetic sequences specific for infective organisms is an emerging technology that offers the advantages of rapid identification combined with high sensitivity and specificity.[54] One group of investigators adopted a procedure that was able to detect as few as 10 bacilli per sample with high accuracy, including detecting *M tuberculosis* in peripheral blood of two of four AIDS patients. All specimens negative by culture were negative by PCR. The only specimens positive by PCR but culture-negative were from a patient who was on a three-drug antituberculous regimen, following a smear-positive gastric aspirate.[55] A second group has identified a DNA sequence that is highly specific for *M tuberculosis* and *M bovis* but not cross-reactive with pathogenic atypical mycobacteria.[56] Clinical studies with this sequence should be forthcoming.

Treatment of Tuberculosis

Historically, the treatment of TB consisted of nutritional replenishment and rest in a specialized sanitarium where a prolonged respite from the stress and pollution of day-to-day life was felt to be therapeutic. In the absence of effective chemotherapeutic agents for almost half a century, the cornerstone of treatment was the obliteration of the pulmonary tuberculous cavity through surgical intervention. Procedures included pneumoperitoneum, pneumothorax, thoracoplasty, and plombage.[18,57]

The chemotherapeutic era of TB treatment was heralded by the application of streptomycin (STM) to the treatment of TB. The effect of this therapy was beneficial, often in a dramatic way, on pulmonary disease; however, extrapulmonary disease continued to be progressive and, when involving the meninges and pericardium, was usually fatal. Over the next several years, it was demonstrated that resistance to STM quickly evolved with single drug therapy and, for this reason, STM was combined with paraaminosalicylic acid (PAS) in an attempt to reduce drug resistance. STM was limited by the necessity for a parenteral route of injection, generally intramuscular and PAS by its unpalatability and side effects. In 1952, isoniazid (INH) was first introduced into the TB armamentarium. With the advent of combination chemotherapy with INH, STM, and/

The major development of the last decade has been the addition of pyrazinamide (PZA) to INH- and RIF- containing regimens.

or PAS, TB was, for the first time, a routinely curable disease. The use of these drugs continues to be the foundation of effective therapy; this was a difficult task, however, as effective therapy required 18–24 months of compliance. In 1970, rifampin (RIF) came into general use, and was recognized as a drug equal to INH in efficacy of anti-TB therapy. The combination of these two tuberculocidal drugs led to studies that demonstrated that 9 months of INH and RIF were of equal or of greater efficacy than 18–24 months of INH and STM.[18,58–60]

The major development of the last decade has been the addition of pyrazinamide (PZA) to INH- and RIF-containing regimens, enabling an intensive four-drug INH-, RIF-, PZA-containing regimen to be given for 2 months, followed by 4 months of maintenance therapy with INH and RIF, which has achieved equal or greater efficacy with a very low rate of relapse.[58,59,61–63]

Additional attempts to further shorten the duration of therapy involving 3- and 4-month regimens have shown some promise. In Arkansas, in smear-negative and culture-negative cases that had positive tuberculin tests and compatible chest radiograph abnormalities, 4 months of INH/RIF led to relapse rates of approximately 1% in one series.[64] Another study in Hong Kong involving patients with negative AFB smears but positive cultures examined relapse rates in INH or STM-sensitive cases (2%) or resistant cases (8%). The authors stated that 4-month chemotherapy is now routinely employed in AFB negative cases. Three-month therapy led to an unacceptably high rate of relapse.[65]

The rationale for combination drug treatment of TB is broadly based on two concepts—the targeting of different populations of mycobacteria according to their metabolic and reproductive activity and surrounding milieu, and that of seeking to prevent the emergence of drug-resistant organisms. In any given tuberculous infection within the body, the TB population is thought to comprise three distinct groups: the first group consists of rapidly dividing

TABLE 1   Site of Action of Anti-TB Drugs

	Cavities	Caseous Material	Intracellular (Macrophage)
INH	+ +	+ +	+ +
Rifampin	+ +	+ +	+ +
Pyrazinamide	—	—	+ +
Ethambutol	+	+	+
Streptomycin	+ +	—	—

INH, isoniazid

bacteria that occur within the pulmonary cavity, which is felt to be a favorable environment with a high oxygen tension and a neutral pH; a second group of organisms exists in the somewhat hypoxic acidic environment of solid caseous parenchymal material; and a third population, still more metabolically inactive, exists within the unfavorable acidic environment of the activated macrophage.[18,59,66] A schema of the site of action of antituberculous chemotherapeutic agents is shown in Table 1.

Antimicrobial Resistance

In addition to the environmental milieu and metabolic state of the mycobacterial organisms, resistance plays a crucial role in determining appropriate drug therapy. It is felt that genetically resistant mutants occur in the different chemotherapeutic agents with the frequency of 10^{-6}–10^{-8} organisms. Because cavities contain between 10^8 and 10^{11} TB organisms per gram of tissue, there are sufficient bacteria to permit an emergent strain to be selected by single-drug therapy. Within noncavitary parenchymal disease, it is felt that 10^4–10^5 mycobacteria exist per gram of tissue; this would be below the threshold statistically necessary to predict the presence of a resistant population.

Primary drug resistance is defined as that which occurs in a previously untreated patient. Secondary drug resistance is defined as resistance that develops within a patient while on treatment for TB. The most important factors that increase the risk of drug resistance include: previous treatment for TB, birth or recent residence in a geographic area associated with a high rate of TB and drug resistance, such as Southeast Asia or Africa, residence within a country associated with increased risk of resistant organisms, and recent exposure to a known case of drug-resistant TB. Secondary drug resistance correlates primarily with selection of an improper regimen, for example, use of a single agent for active disease or a single tuberculocidal agent combined with a static agent for cavitary disease, or in most cases, a lack of compliance on the patient's part. Patients who take all of their medications as prescribed and then, for reasons of toxicity or poor compliance, stop all of the medications at the same time, generally are repopulated with sensitive organisms. However, if the patient stops the medications in a staggered fashion, or takes the medications on an intermittent basis, the chances for development of secondary drug resistance increase dramatically.

In the United States, the prevalence of resistance to INH or STM is approximately 7–10%; however, this varies widely with geographic location, with much higher rates being recorded along the Mexican border and in areas

In addition to the environmental milieu and metabolic state of the mycobacterial organisms, resistance plays a crucial role in determining appropriate drug therapy.

The prevalence of resistance to INH or STM in the United States varies widely with geographic location, but is approximately 7–10%.

where recent immigrants from countries with high rates of drug-resistant TB relocate. These countries tend to be ones where antituberculous medication can be bought over the counter and administered in an unsupervised fashion. For example, the rate of drug resistance is very high in oriental wives of U.S. servicemen coming from countries such as Korea and the Philippines.

Typically, INH, RIF, PZA, STM, and ethambutol (EMB) are referred to as primary, or first-line therapeutic agents, and ethionamide (ETH), PAS, cycloserine, capreomycin, kanamycin, amikacin, and thiacetazone are referred to as second-line agents. [18,58,59,66]

Isoniazid (INH Isonicotinic Acid Hydrozide)

Isoniazid acts by inhibiting mycolic acid synthesis and oxygen-dependent metabolic processes of *M tuberculosis*. The drug is well absorbed after oral administration and is distributed throughout the body tissues, including the central nervous system. Isoniazid is bactericidal for TB in all tissues including caseous foci, macrophages, and the meninges. It is metabolized in the liver by the P450 microsomal enzyme system involving both acetylation and oxidation. Acetylation is genetically determined, and rapid acetylators, predominantly in the oriental population, tend to have serum concentrations significantly lower than those of slow acetylators seen more commonly in caucasians. The relationship of acetylator status to development of INH hepatotoxicity is controversial, with studies showing an increased prevalence in both the slow and rapid acetylator groups. INH-induced hepatitis is clearly age-related, with an increase in incidence accompanying advancing age, as shown in Table 2. INH-induced hepatitis is discussed in more detail in the section on INH and Rifampin Hepatotoxicity. The other major toxicity commonly seen with isoniazid therapy is a peripheral neuropathy secondary to

TABLE 2   Age-related Incidence of (INH) Hepatotoxicity

Age (years)	Hepatotoxicity Rate (%)	
<20	Rare	
20–34	0.3	
35–49	1.2	Overall, 1–2%
≥50	2.3	
>65	~4	
INH + Rifampin:	4–8%	
PZA:	No additional hepatotoxicity	

INH, isoniazid; PZA, pyrazinamide

pyridoxine (vitamin B_6) depletion, which can be prevented by the administration of 50 mg/day of pyridoxine. This is especially important in patients who have underlying peripheral neuropathy for other reasons, such as diabetes, uremia, or demyelinating conditions. Coexistent pyridoxine deficiency may also be seen with increased frequency in alcoholics, patients with end-stage renal disease, those who are chronically malnourished, persons with cancer, or pregnant women. Unusual toxicities of INH include seizures, development of an ANA-positive state, and rarely drug-induced lupus erythematosus. Other rare toxicities include skin eruptions, psychosis, and Dupuytren's contractures.

Rifampin (RIF)

Rifampin is an inhibitor of deoxyribonucleic acid (DNA)-dependent RNA polymerase, which was introduced into clinical trials in 1966 and adopted for widespread use in 1970. Like INH, it is bactericidal in very low concentrations with a rapid onset of action. It is well absorbed after oral administration and distributed throughout the body including the CSF. Minor adverse reactions include gastrointestinal (GI) intolerance and transient liver function abnormalities. The incidence of hepatotoxicity is increased at least four-fold when INH and RIF are given concurrently. An unusual and distinctive toxic reaction occurs primarily in individuals who receive intermittent therapy (for example, twice weekly or less often with doses larger than 600 mg/day). This reaction appears to be immunologically mediated and can include hemolytic anemia, development of acute renal failure, and thrombocytopenia. It should be emphasized that this side effect is very rare when rifampin is administered in daily doses. RIF also stains body fluids an orange color and can stain soft contact lenses. It is a potent inducer of the P450-mixed oxidative enzymes, which can increase catabolism of corticosteroids, oral contraceptives, coumadin, ketoconazole, dilantin, and cyclosporine. Unwanted pregnancies in users of oral contraceptives, unexpectedly low dilantin levels in patients being treated for seizures, as well as unexpectedly low cyclosporine levels in patients receiving immunosuppressive therapy have all been noted.

INH and Rifampin Hepatotoxicity

Symptomatic INH hepatitis occurs in 1–2% of all patients treated with INH. It is felt that the toxic moiety represents a byproduct of oxidative metabolism rather than acet-

The rate of INH hepatotoxicity increased dramatically in patients treated with INH and RIF together.

ylation. In addition, the rate of INH hepatotoxicity increases dramatically in patients treated with INH and RIF together.

The risk of frank hepatitis is increased four-fold, and elevations of liver function tests less than five times above the normal range have occurred in 10–20% of patients. When patients develop frank symptomatic hepatitis as manifested by nausea, vomiting, and jaundice, the risk of death is 6–12%. In addition, it appears that with combined INH/RIF the onset of jaundice occurs earlier, often within 1–3 weeks of the onset of treatment. This may be due to an acceleration of INH oxidation and accumulation of toxic metabolites resulting from the effects of RIF on the hepatic P450 microsomal oxidase system.

Routine baseline biochemical testing of transaminase levels is no longer recommended.

Routine baseline biochemical testing of transaminase levels are no longer recommended. In general, most authorities recommend that patients be counseled to discontinue therapy immediately upon development of suspicious symptoms, such as nausea, vomiting, anorexia, scleral icterus, or jaundice, and to report to the TB clinic for transaminase determination and clinical evaluation. If symptoms are accompanied by elevations of greater than or equal to five times the baseline level of liver transaminases, then drug toxicity is likely. After symptoms have abated and enzymes have returned to baseline, drugs are reintroduced one at a time starting with one-half the dosage, and the hepatic enzymes are monitored closely. Given this process, the offending drug can often be identified and therapy appropriately adjusted. When recurrent hepatitis occurs and is attributable to INH (eg, in a non-RIF regimen), it is appropriate to proceed with the use of RIF and two companion drugs to take the place of INH. When hepa-

---

TABLE 3   Algorithm for Management of Anti-TB Medication-associated Hepatotoxicity

Initial Regimen	Subsequent Regimen*
INH + RIF + PZA + EMB	→ INH + RIF ($\frac{1}{2}$ dose) + PZA + EMB or INH + PZA + EMB + STM
INH + STM + EMB	→ RIF + STM + EMB
INH + RIF	→ INH + STM + EMB or INH + PZA ($\times$ 18 mo)
INH + RIF (resistant to INH)	→ RIF + STM + EMB or RIF + PZA ($\times$ 18 mo)

INH, isoniazid; RIF, rifampin; PZA, pyrazinamide; EMB, ethambutol; STM, streptomycin
* Allow LFTs to normalize prior to reinstituting therapy unless emergent treatment indicated. Once hepatotoxicity (transaminases $\geq 5 \times$ normal) has occurred, one should follow sequential LFTs.

totoxicity accompanies the addition of RIF to INH, it is appropriate to proceed with INH plus two companion drugs to take the place of RIF. When RIF is omitted from chemotherapy, it is necessary to continue therapy for a longer period of time, for example for 18–24 months, rather than the standard 6–9 months. Once hepatotoxicity has occurred, it is important to monitor liver function tests and to increase dosages gradually. In cases in which hepatotoxicity occurs and INH resistance has been found, one would restart RIF plus two companion drugs. An algorithm for management of anti-TB medication-associated hepatotoxicity is shown in Table 3.

When RIF is omitted from chemotherapy, therapy must be continued for a longer period of time.

Pyrazinamide (PZA)

Pyrazinamide, like INH, is a nicotinic acid derivative that was first investigated in the 1950s but was felt to be prohibitively hepatotoxic. However, it was initially given at a dose of 40–50 mg/kg/day. In the 1970s, interest was revived in PZA because of its lack of toxicity at a dose of 30–35 mg/kg/day and its important role in short-course chemotherapy regimens. PZA is not found to increase the risk of hepatotoxicity beyond that encountered with INH and RIF. It is metabolized by the liver and should be given at a reduced dosage or avoided altogether in severe hepatic failure. A major metabolite, pyrazinoic acid, is excreted by the kidney, and a dosage modification is necessary in renal failure. In addition, this metabolite interferes with renal tubular uric acid secretion, leading to an incidence greater than 50% of hyperuricemia during treatment, usually asymptomatic. In a minority of patients, mild arthralgias will ensue, and in rarer patients, precipitation of frank gout has been seen. PZA is active only in pH 5.6 or less, an acid environment found within macrophage phagolysosomes.

Ethambutol (EMB)

Ethambutol acts by inhibition of RNA synthesis within *M tuberculosis*. It is 80% bioavailable after oral administration and is widely distributed, including across inflamed meninges. In addition, it is well tolerated and at lower doses, nontoxic. Since it is excreted unchanged in the urine, in the presence of renal failure a dosage reduction is necessary. Hyperuricemia can occur due to impaired renal excretion of uric acid, as is seen in PZA. With higher doses of 25 mg/kg/day, one may see a retrobulbar neuritis that is first manifested as decreasing color vision, progressing to

EMB is frequently used as the fourth drug in short-course chemotherapeutic regimens or as a companion drug with INH for individuals who have either RIF-resistant organisms or are intolerant of RIF.

decreasing visual acuity. It is largely reversible if discontinued early. EMB is frequently used as the fourth drug in short-course chemotherapeutic regimens or as a companion drug with INH for individuals who have either RIF-resistant organisms or are intolerant of RIF.

Streptomycin (STM)

Streptomycin (STM) is the least nephrotoxic of aminoglycoside antibiotics; however, vestibular toxicity soon became apparent, as did the emergence of resistance. Although other aminoglycosides exhibit marginally greater activity against TB than STM, its low cost and therapeutic index combined with its long track record have made this the most widely used drug of its class. Because it is primarily excreted by the kidneys, a major dosage reduction is necessary in the presence of renal failure. In addition, it appears to be mainly active in cavitary disease with a much lower activity in the setting of intracellular bacteria within acidic environments. Another major drawback of STM and aminoglycosides is that they do not cross the blood brain barrier.

Other aminoglycosides that may see greater use include capreomycin and amikacin, especially as salvage therapy for treatment of drug-resistant strains. Amikacin has excellent antituberculous activity; however, its extremely high cost has limited its use in the United States and essentially prohibited its use worldwide.

Second-line Bacteriostatic Antituberculous Medications

Paraaminosalicylic acid (PAS) is an antifolate drug. Its unpleasant taste and GI side effects led to very poor patient compliance. In one study, urinary screening for PAS found it present in only 58% of the patients for whom it had been prescribed.

Ethionimide is a synthetic derivative of isonicotinic acid. It is well absorbed after oral administration and is distributed into the CSF. Side effects include GI irritation, reversible hepatotoxicity, peripheral neuropathy, and psychosis. Like INH, some of its side effects are prevented by the coadministration of pyridoxine.

Cycloserine interferes with cell-wall synthesis of *M tuberculosis*. It is well absorbed after oral administration and is distributed within the brain and CSF. Unfortunately, it has potential for lowering the seizure threshold and has also been associated with toxic psychosis.

Investigational drugs include ansamycin, some beta-lactamase resistant cephalosporins, potentially other beta-lactam drugs combined with clavulinic acid, and a wide variety of quinolones. In the case of many of these newer drugs, their potential usefulness has been limited by their high cost and the rapid emergence of resistance.

Therapeutic Regimens for Treatment of Tuberculosis

In the 1970s, the combination of INH with EMB with or without STM given for a period of 18–24 months led to successful therapeutic outcome and a relapse rate of less than 5%, which is now considered the gold standard for an acceptable treatment regimen. With the widespread use of RIF, it became apparent that INH and RIF, with or without EMB or STM for the first 2 months, for a total duration of 9 months, gave an equivalent success and relapse rate. This was adopted as the standard treatment regimen by the American Thoracic Society in 1980. The current standard regimen, which has evolved over the course of the 1980s, based largely on work initially done by the British Medical Research Council in the Orient and more recently replicated in the United States, is for treatment with INH, RIF, PZA, and either STM or EMB for 2 months of induction therapy, followed by INH and RIF for 4 months of consolidation therapy.[59,61–63,65,66] This regimen, which is given as a daily dose for the first 2 months, can be given either daily or twice weekly during the last 4 months of INH and RIF consolidative therapy. Both regimens have shown a relapse rate of less than 5%. In addition, a regimen giving INH and RIF daily for 2 months, followed by twice weekly for another 7 months, has an acceptable rate of success.[60] In this regimen, the twice-weekly dosage of INH is increased to 900 mg.

It appears that the key element in the evolution of this 6-month therapeutic regimen is the inclusion of PZA. Its highly bactericidal activity has led to unexpected successes for limited disease with as little as 2, 3, or 4 months of therapy, especially in the setting of smear-negative and culture-negative diseases.[65] In addition, by incorporating four drugs into the initial therapeutic regimen, one minimizes the chances of an unsuccessful outcome on the basis of primary drug resistance. A summary of acceptable antituberculous drug regimens is shown in Table 4.

The current standard regimen is for treatment with INH, RIF, PZA, and either STM or EMB for 2 months of induction therapy, followed by INH and RIF for 4 months of consolidation therapy.

It appears that the key element in the evolution of this 6-month therapeutic regimen is the inclusion of PZA.

TABLE 4   Comparison of Anti-TB Regimens

1980 Standard Regimen	INH/RIF/EMB or STM × 2 mo → INH/RIF × 7 mo (daily or twice weekly)
Current Standard Regimen	INH/RIF/PZA and STM or EMB × 2 mo → INH/RIF × 4 mo
INH—Resistance	INH/RIF/PZA/STM × ≥9 mo
STM—Resistance	INH/RIF/PZA/EMB × ≥9 mo
RIF—Resistance	INH/EMB/STM × 2 mo → INH/ EMB × 16 mo
Multiply Resistant	(eg, INH/RIF/STM) Substitute 2 static or 2nd-line (or retreatment) drugs for each cidal drug deleted, based on additional drug sensitivity testing × 18–24 mo

Strict compliance must be assured.
INH, isoniazid; RIF, rifampin; EMB, ethambutol; STM, streptomycin; PZA, pyrazinamide

Follow-up Study of Patients Undergoing Anti-TB Therapy

Ideally, therapy should be guided by drug-susceptibility testing, and therefore, every effort should be made to obtain a specific diagnosis and positive culture. In smear-negative cases, multiple (eg, five) sputum specimens should be obtained if possible, and one should consider bronchoscopy if expectorated sputa are smear-negative. In severely ill patients, treatment should be initiated immediately and an attempt at specific diagnosis pursued.

During treatment, some experts advocate checking sputa at 1 month of therapy and at 2–4-week intervals thereafter to document conversion of a smear-positive to a smear-negative status and conversion of cultures from positive to negative.[59] Others recommend smears and cultures at 2, 4, and 6 months of treatment.[18] In general, INH- and RIF-containing regimens will show conversion by 2 months. If sputa remain culture-positive after 4 months of treatment, drug resistance is likely.

Patients receiving INH-containing regimens should be instructed about symptoms of hepatitis, although in normal hosts, it is no longer recommended to monitor transaminase levels routinely during therapy. Individuals receiving both INH and RIF, especially if they are alcoholics or if they have chronic liver disease, may be followed with transaminase levels. It is controversial whether chronic liver disease, such as chronic hepatitis B surface antigenemia or chronic hepatitis B, predisposes to an increased incidence of INH hepatotoxicity.[67]

If sputa remain culture-positive after 4 months of treatment, drug resistance is likely.

Patients receiving EMB should be questioned at regular intervals regarding visual symptoms and a baseline visual acuity, and red-green color testing should be performed in those receiving higher doses, such as 25 mg/kg/day.

Individuals receiving aminoglycosides should have baseline audiograms and should be questioned about high-frequency hearing loss and for symptoms of vestibulitis.

Many authors feel that after completion of therapy follow-up study with a clinical evaluation, sputum, and chest radiograph should be undertaken every 3–6 months for a period of 1–2 years. More prolonged follow-up study is no longer routinely advocated; however, those who were slow to convert from positive to negative, those who were suspected of poor compliance, immunocompromised patients, and those with very extensive disease may be followed more closely.

Surveillance of Patient Compliance During Therapy

It is important to remember that compliance is one of the keys to effective drug therapy in the treatment of TB. This should be ensured by frequent interviews with the patient, checking attendance at clinic appointments, picking up of drugs, surprise pill counts, and random examination of the urine for orange color of RIF. In patients thought to be noncompliant, direct ingestion of drugs under supervision should be carried out. Administration of injectable drugs such as STM also helps to ensure compliance. Twice-weekly administration of drugs also facilitates direct supervision. Public health nurses perform the key roles of contact evaluation, tuberculin testing, and critical follow-up study of patients during the period of treatment.

Patient compliance is one of the keys to effective drug therapy in the treatment of TB.

Surgical Treatment of TB Complications

Today the indications for surgical therapy in TB are the presence of persistent or drug-resistant disease, treatment failure as associated with resectable cavitary lesions, disease occurring in a patient with a resectable lesion who is unable to cooperate with chemotherapeutic treatment, presence of bronchiectasis, presence of severe hemoptysis, and suspicion of possible neoplasm.[18,57,68] In one recent review of surgical treatment of TB complications,[68] in many patients, there was more than one complication necessitating surgery—the most common complications were persistent disease in 33%, bronchiectasis in 50%, and hemoptysis in 67%. Of note, in a series of 24 patients, the average estimated operative blood loss was 1,150 mL and the overall complication rate of surgery was 48%, with 17% having major complications, including bronchopleural fistula, empyema, and pneumonia.

Retreatment

The key concepts involved in retreatment of patients with TB are to base therapy upon susceptibility testing and to ensure strict compliance with the prescribed regimen.

The key concepts involved in retreatment of patients with TB are to base therapy upon susceptibility testing and to ensure strict compliance with the prescribed regimen, since there is a finite number of antituberculous drugs and the loss of additional drugs to which the organism is susceptible is potentially disastrous. Most patients with resistant organisms should be treated by individuals with expertise in management of these patients. As mentioned before, if sputum cultures remain positive after more than 4–5 months of treatment, in general, resistance will be present. A relapse occurring promptly after sputum conversion has occurred often indicates that the drugs have been stopped too soon, usually by the patient. If the patient has stopped all drugs concomitantly, often the organisms will still be susceptible. However, if the drugs have been stopped in a haphazard or erratic fashion, organisms will develop resistance. For treatment of resistant organisms, a three- or four-drug combination is recommended, with the substitution of at least one tuberculocidal drug and the addition of one second-line drug.[18,26,59,59] When organisms are resistant to INH, RIF, STM, and PZA, one should consider adding four second-line drugs with the addition of INH at a higher dose of 15 mg/kg/day, which still retains inhibitory effects.[18] A summary of recommended dosages of different antituberculous drugs is found in Table 5.

For treatment of resistant organisms, a three- or four-drug combination is recommended, with the substitution of at least one tuberculocidal drug and the addition of one second-line drug.

TABLE 5   Standard Dosages of Anti-TB Medications

First-line Agents		Second-line Agents	
INH	300 mg qd or 900 mg 2×/wk (in children, 10 mg/kg/day up to 300 mg)	PAS	200 mg/kg/day (10–12 g qd)
RIF	600 mg qd (in children, 15 mg/kg/day up to 600 mg)	Ethionamide	10–15 mg/kg/day (500–1,000 mg qd)
PZA	25–35 mg/kg/day	Cycloserine	15 mg/kg/day (750–1,000 mg qd)
STM	1 g qd (500 mg in elderly ≥ 65) (in children, 20 mg/kg/day)	Kanamycin	0.5 gm qd or 1.0 g 3–4 ×/wk
EMB	15–25 mg/kg/day (in children, 15 mg/kg/day)	Amikacin	7.5 mg/day (500 mg qd)
		Capreomycin	15 mg/kg/day (1 g/day)
		Ciprofloxacin	500 mg bid or 750 mg qd

INH, isoniazid; RIF, rifampin; PZA, pyrazinamide; STM, streptomycin; EMB, ethambutol; PAS, paraaminosal cylic acid

Chemoprophylactic Preventive Therapy

As mentioned in the section on diagnostic studies, the standard historical criterion for a positive PPD is ≥10 mm in induration; that has been changed to state that for individuals who are HIV positive, or otherwise immunocompromised, ≥5 mm of induration is now considered positive. It is recommended that all HIV-positive patients have their PPD status assessed and that all TB patients have their HIV status assessed.[4] The American Thoracic Society and Centers for Disease Control recommended the following groups for preventive therapy:

1. Household members and other close contacts of patients with infectious TB with a positive tuberculin test and no previous history of reaction in the past. Contacts under the age of 4 years with a negative TB skin test should be given preventive therapy for 3 months and assessed again after 3 months with tuberculin tests; if negative, therapy is discontinued. Otherwise, the full course is completed.

2. Newly infected persons, tuberculin converters within the last 2 years.

3. Persons with a history of inadequately treated TB.

4. Persons with a significant reaction (≥15 mm induration) and a stable abnormal chest radiograph.

5. Positive tuberculin reaction-associated risk factors, such as silicosis, diabetes mellitus, prolonged therapy with steroids greater than or equal to 1 month in duration, immunosuppressive therapy, hematologic, and reticuloendothelial malignancy, AIDS or HIV positivity, end-stage renal disease, and clinical conditions leading to rapid weight loss and chronic malnutrition.

6. Tuberculin skin test reactors under 35 years of age.

Preventative therapy consists of INH, 300 mg/day for adults for a period of 6–12 months, with the former employed in most cases. Therapy in children is for 10–14 mg/kg, not to exceed 300 mg/day. It is recommended that clinical monitoring for symptoms is adequate, and hepatic transaminases should not routinely be checked. The supply of medication to the patient should be limited to 1 month at a time. The patients should be advised to discontinue therapy should they develop nausea, vomiting, diarrhea or jaundice, and to report to their physician for evaluation.

Although there are no data available for prophylaxis of exposure to INH-resistant cases, it is thought that RIF, 600 mg daily for 12 months, is the most reasonable course.

Control of infectivity is best achieved by administering specific antituberculous therapy.

Although there are no data available for prophylaxis of exposure to INH-resistant cases, it is felt that RIF, 600 mg daily for 12 months, is the most reasonable course.[70] Studies have varied as to the efficacy of TB chemoprophylaxis in this setting, with reported rates of between 60% and 85%.[71]

Prevention and Infection Control

Transmission of TB occurs through airborne spread of bacilli in aerosols. This places contacts of infected persons, such as family members, hospital personnel, and other close contacts, at risk for secondary spread of the infection. Control of infectivity is best done by administering specific antituberculous therapy, generally rendering the patient noncommunicable in 2–3 weeks if accompanied by a clinical and bacteriologic (fewer organisms by smear) response. Hospitalization is required for seriously ill patients and for those with social reasons that preclude therapy at home. Smear-positive persons who are hospitalized should be isolated in a private room with negative-pressure ventilation. Ultraviolet light may aid in decontaminating the air in the room by killing airborne bacilli. Persons entering the room must wear a mask or particulate respirator and employ proper handwashing techniques to prevent secondary transmission.[73] Persons who are on an appropriate therapeutic regimen for 2–3 weeks with a clinical and bacteriologic response are probably no longer infectious.[72,73] Caution should be exercised, however, when such a person is put in a room with another patient, particularly if the other patient is immunocompromised.[73]

Investigation of cases contacts should be conducted to detect asymptomatic transmission. Mantoux (PPD) skin tests should be placed as soon as possible for PPD negative contacts. All contact with a negative test should be retested 10 weeks from the time of exposure. The incubation period from infection to a positive reaction or identifiable primary disease is usually 4–12 weeks. Positive reactors should be referred for appropriate therapy. Chest radiographs are performed on all skin-test-positive persons to detect asymptomatic primary disease. The majority of persons infected who develop clinical disease do so in the first 6–12 months after infection. Those at greatest risk of developing primary disease are children less than 3 years of age, adolescents and young adults, and the elderly. Thus it is imperative to identify infected contacts to decrease the likelihood of further spread of TB as well as to decrease the incidence of symptomatic disease through the utilization of postconversion chemoprophylaxis. All cases of TB in-

The majority of infected persons who develop clinical disease do so in the first 6–12 months after infection. Those at greatest risk of developing primary disease are children less than 3 years of age, adolescents and young adults, and the elderly.

fection, regardless of symptoms, should be reported to the local health department so that surveillance, follow-up study and treatment methods can be implemented in a coordinated manner.

The requirement for periodic repeat PPD skin testing for hospital personnel depends upon the risk of exposure. This risk is dependent upon the number and location of tuberculous patients admitted to the hospital and the prevalence of TB in the community. Hospitals with a low exposure risk may screen annually, whereas other hospitals or areas of a hospital with a high exposure risk may choose to implement this practice semiannually, particularly with personnel who perform high-risk procedures (bronchoscopy, sputum induction, aerosol treatments). Periodic chest radiographs for employees who have completed an adequate course of prophylaxis or treatment are not indicated.[73] Due to recent reports of outbreaks of pulmonary TB in the elderly, especially those residing in nursing homes,[16] periodic testing of these populations may also be indicated for those persons who are not previously known to be PPD positive.

The requirement for periodic repeat PPD skin testing for hospital personnel depends upon the risk of exposure.

References

1. Murray JF: The white plague: down and out, or up and coming? Am Rev Respir Dis 140:1788, 1989

2. Reider HL, Cauthen GM, Kelly GD et al: State of the art/review: tuberculosis in the United States. Riesenberg D, Section Editor. JAMA 262:385, 1989

3. Selwyn PA, Hartel D, Lewis VA et al: A prospective study of the risk of tuberculosis among intravenous drug users with human immunodeficiency virus infection. N Engl J Med 320:545, 1989

4. Centers for Disease Control: Tuberculosis and human immunodeficiency virus infection: recommendations of the Advisory Committee for the Elimination of Tuberculosis (ACET). MMWR 38:236, 1989

5. Centers for Disease Control: Tuberculosis and acquired immunodeficiency syndrome—Florida. MMRW 35:587, 1986

6. Centers for Disease Control: Tuberculosis and acquired immunodeficiency syndrome—New York City. MMWR 36:785, 1987

7. Centers for Disease Control: Supplement: A strategic plan for the elimination of tuberculosis in the United States. MMWR 38(Suppl-3):1, 1989

8. Stead WW, Senner JW, Reddick WT, Lofgren JP: Racial differences in susceptibility of infection by *Mycobacterium tuberculosis*. N Engl J Med 322:422, 1990

9. Crowle AJ, Elkins N: Relative permissiveness of macrophages from black and white people for virulent tubercule bacilli. Infect Immun 58:632, 1990

10. Centers for Disease Control: Update: tuberculosis elimination—United States. MMWR 39:153, 1990

11. Centers for Disease Control: Tuberculosis Control Division: Tuberculosis in the United States, 1981–84. Centers for Disease Control, Atlanta, 3, 1986

12. Stead WW: Special problems in tuberculosis: tuberculosis in the elderly and in residents of nursing homes, correctional facilities, long-term care hospitals, mental hospitals, shelters for the homeless, and jails. Clin Chest Med 10:397, 1989

13. Centers for Disease Control: *Mycobacterium tuberculosis* transmission in a health clinic—Florida. MMWR 38:256, 1989

14. Centers for Disease Control: Tuberculosis in developing countries. MMWR 39:561, 1990

15. Stead WW, Lofgren JP, Warren E et al: Tuberculosis as an endemic and nosocomial infection among the elderly in nursing homes. N Engl J Med 312:1483, 1985

16. Nardell E, McInnis B, Thomas B et al: Exogenous reinfection with tuberculosis in a shelter for the homeless. N Engl J Med 315:1570, 1986

17. Bass JB Jr, Farer LS, Hopewell PC et al: Diagnostic standards and classification of tuberculosis. Am Rev Respir Dis 142:725, 1990

18. Desprez RM, Heim CR: Mycobacterium tuberculosis. p. 1877. In Mandell GL, Douglas RG, Bennett JE (eds): Principles and practice of infectious diseases. Third ed., Churchill Livingstone, New York, 1990

19. Heffner JE, Strange C, Sahn SA: The impact of respiratory failure on the diagnosis of tuberculosis. Arch Intern Med 148:403, 1988

20. Barnes PF, Verdegem TD, Vachon LA: Chest roentgenogram in pulmonary tuberculosis. Chest 94:316, 1988

21. Pitchenik AE, Rubinson HA: The radiographic appearance of tuberculosis in patients with the acquired immune deficiency syndrome (AIDS) and Pre-AIDS. Am Rev Respir Dis 131:393, 1985

22. Chang S, Lee P, Perry P: Lower lung field tuberculosis. Chest 91:230, 1987

23. Van den Brande PM, Van de Mierop F, Verbeken EK: Endobronchial tuberculosis in the elderly. Arch Intern Med 150:2105, 1990

24. Anntoniskis D, Amin K, Barnes PF: Pleuritis as a manifestation of reactivation tuberculosis. Am J Med 4:447, 1990

25. McClement JH, Christenson LC: Clinical forms of tuberculosis. p. 1288. In Fishman A (ed): Pulmonary diseases and disorders. McGraw-Hill, New York, 1980

26. Mangura BT, Reichman LB: Pulmonary tuberculosis. p. 528. In Pennington JE (ed): Respiratory infections: diagnosis and management. Second Edition. Raven Press, New York, 1988

27. Stead WW, To T: The significance of the tuberculin skin test in elderly persons. Ann Intern Med 107:837, 1987

28. Alvarez S, Kasprzyk DR, Freundl M: Two-stage skin testing for tuberculosis in a domiciliary population. Am Rev Respir Dis 136:1193, 1987

29. Perez-Stable EJ, Flaherty D, Schecter G et al: Conversion and reversion of tuberculin reactions in nursing home residents. Am Rev Respir Dis 137:801, 1988

30. Gordin F, Slutkin G: The validity of acid-fast smears in the diagnosis of pulmonary tuberculosis. Arch Pathol Lab Med 114:1025, 1990

31. Berean K, Roberts FJ: The reliability of acid-fast stained smears of gastric aspirate specimens. Tubercle 69:205, 1988

32. Klotz SA, Penn RL: Acid-fast staining of urine and gastric contents is an excellent indicator of mycobacterial disease. Am Rev Respir Dis 136:1197, 1987

33. Fisher JF, Ganapathy M, Edwards BH, Newman CL: Utility of Gram's and giemsa stains in the diagnosis of pulmonary tuberculosis. Am Rev Respir Dis 141:511, 1990

34. Raja A, Machicao AR, Morrissey AB et al: Specific detection of *Mycobacterium tuberculosis* in radiometric cultures by using an immunoassay for antigen 5. J Infect Dis 158:468, 1988

35. de Garcia J, Curull V, Vidal R et al: Diagnostic value of bronchoalveolar lavage in suspected pulmonary tuberculosis. Chest 93:329, 1988

36. Kim TCH, Blackman RS, Heatwole KM et al: Acid-fast bacilli in sputum smears of patients with pulmonary tuberculosis. Am Rev Respir Dis 129:264, 1984

37. Styblo K, Rouillon A: Estimated global incidence of smear-positive pulmonary tuberculosis. Unreliability of officially reported figures on tuberculosis. Bull Int Union Tuberc Lung Dis 56:118, 1981

38. Charpin D, Herbault H, Gevaudan MJ et al: Value of ELISA using A60 antigen in the diagnosis of active pulmonary tuberculosis. Am Rev Respir Dis 142:380, 1990

39. Espitia C, Cervera I, Gonzalez R, Mancilla R: A 38-kD *Mycobacterium tuberculosis* antigen associated with infection: its isolation and serologic evaluation. Clin Exp Immunol 77:373, 1989

40. Wilkins EGL, Ivanyi J: Potential value of serology for diagnosis of extrapulmonary tuberculosis. Lancet 336:641, 1990

41. Sada DE, Ferguson LE, Daniel TM: An ELISA for the serodiagnosis of tuberculosis using a 30,000-Da native antigen of *Mycobacterium tuberculosis*. J Infect Dis 162:928, 1990

42. Chan SL, Reggiardo Z, Daniel TM et al: Serodiagnosis of tuberculosis using an ELISA with antigen 5 and a hemagglutination assay with glycolipid antigens. Am Rev Respir Dis 142:385, 1990

43. Larsson L, Mardh PA, Odham G: Detection of tuberculostearic acid in mycobacteria and nocardiae by gas chromatography and mass spectrometry using selected ion monitoring. J Chromatogr 163:221, 1979

44. French GL, Chan CY, Cheung SW, Oo KT: Diagnosis of pulmonary tuberculosis by detection of tuberculostearic acid in sputum by using gas chromatography-mass spectrometry with selected ion monitoring. J Infect Dis 156:356, 1987

45. Pang JA, Chan HS, Chan CY et al: A tuberculostearic acid assay in the diagnosis of sputum smear-negative pulmonary tuberculosis. Ann Intern Med 111:650, 1989

46. Muranishi H, Nakashima M, Isobe R et al: Measurement of tuberculostearic acid in sputa, pleural effusions, and bronchial washings: a clinical evaluation for diagnosis of pulmonary tuberculosis. Diagn Microbiol Infect Dis 13:235, 1990

47. Petterson T, Ojala K, Weber TH: Adenosine deaminase in the diagnosis of pleural effusion. Acta Med Scand 215:299, 1984

48. Ocana I, Martin-Vazquez JM, Segura RM et al: Adenosine deaminase in pleural fluids. Chest 84:51, 1983

49. Perille PE, Kahn K, Finch SC: Serum lysozyme in pulmonary tuberculosis. Am J Med Sci 265:297, 1973

50. Klockars M, Petterson T, Riska H: Pleural fluid lysozyme in human disease. Arch Intern Med 139:73, 1979

51. Verea H, Masa J, Dominguez L et al: Meaning and diagnostic value of determination of pleural fluid lysozyme. Chest 91:342, 1987

52. Asseo P, Tracopoulos GD, Kotsovoulou-Fouskaki V: Lysozyme in pleural effusions and serum. Am J Clin Pathol 78:763, 1982

53. Bueso JF, Hernando HV, Garcia-Buela JP et al: Diagnostic value of simultaneous determination

of pleural adenosine deaminase and pleural lysozyme/serum lysozyme ratio in pleural effusions. Chest 93:303, 1988

54. Saiki RK, Gelfand DH, Stoffel S et al: Primer-directed enzymatic amplification of DNA with thermostable DNA polymerase. Science 239:487, 1988

55. Brisson-Noel A, Gicquel B, Lecossier D et al: Rapid diagnosis of tuberculosis by amplification of mycobacterial DNA in clinical samples. Lancet 2:1069, 1989

56. Eisenach KD, Cave MD, Bates JH, Crawford JT: Polymerase chain reaction amplification of a repetitive DNA sequence specific for *Mycobacterium tuberculosis*. J Infect Dis 161:977, 1990

57. Newman MM: The olden days of surgery for tuberculosis. Ann Thorac Surg 48:161, 1989

58. Grosset JH: Present status of chemotherapy for tuberculosis. Rev Infect Dis 11(Suppl 2):S347, 1989

59. Dutt AK, Stead WW: Tuberculosis in current therapy in infectious diseases. Volume 3, BC Deker, Philadelphia, 1990

60. Slutkin G, Schecter GF, Hopewell PC: The results of 9-month isoniazid-rifampin therapy for pulmonary tuberculosis under program conditions in San Francisco. Am Rev Respir Dis 138:1622, 1988

61. Singapore Tuberculosis Service/British Medical Research Council: Five-year follow-up of a clinical trial of three 6-month regimens of chemotherapy given intermittently in the continuation phase in the treatment of pulmonary tuberculosis. Am Rev Respir Dis 137:1147, 1988

62. Cohn DL, Catlin BJ, Peterson KL et al: A 62-dose, 6-month therapy for pulmonary and extrapulmonary tuberculosis. A twice-weekly, directly observed, and cost-effective regimen. Ann Intern Med 112:407, 1990

63. Combs DL, O'Brien RJ. Geiter LJ: USPHS tuberculosis short-course chemotherapy trial 21: effectiveness, toxicity, and acceptability: the report of final results. Ann Intern Med 112:397, 1990

64. Dutt AK, Moers D, Stead WW: Smear- and culture-negative pulmonary tuberculosis: four-month short-course chemotherapy. Am Rev Respir Dis 139:867, 1989

65. Hong Kong Chest Service/Medical Research Council: A controlled trial of 3-month, 4-month, and 6-month regimens of chemotherapy for sputum-smear-negative pulmonary tuberculosis: results at 5 years. Am Rev Respir Dis 139:871, 1989

66. Alford RH, Manian FA: Current antimicrobial management of tuberculosis. p. 204. In Remington JE, Swartz MN (eds): clinical topics in infectious diseases. Volume 8, McGraw-Hill, New York, 1987

67. Wu JC, Lee SD, Yeh PF et al: Isoniazid-rifampin-induced hepatitis in hepatitis B carriers. Gastroenterology 98:502, 1990

68. Reed CE, Parker EF, Crawford FA Jr: Surgical resection for complications of pulmonary tuberculosis. Ann Thorac Surg 48:165, 1989

69. Davidson PT: Drug resistance and the selection of therapy for tuberculosis. Am Rev Respir Dis 136:255, 1987

70. Centers for Disease Control: Advisory committee for elimination of tuberculosis. The use of preventive therapy for tuberculous infection in the United States. MMWR 39(RR-8):9, 1990

71. International Union Against Tuberculosis Committee on Prophylaxis: Efficacy of various durations of isoniazid preventive therapy for tuberculosis: five years of follow-up in the IVAT trial. Bull WHO 60:555, 1982

72. Benenson AS, Legters LJ et al: Control of communicable diseases in man. 15th ed., American Public Health Association, Washington, DC, 1990

73. Centers for Disease Control: Guidelines for preventing the transmission of tuberculosis in health-care settings, with special focus on HIV-related issues. MMWR 39(RR-17): 7, 1990

74. Sanford JP: Hospital infections. 2nd ed., Little Brown, Boston, 1986

MYCOBACTERIAL DISEASE IN HUMAN IMMUNO-DEFICIENCY VIRUS INFECTION

JEAN A. SMITH, MD

Human immunodeficiency virus (HIV) infection causes a progressive deterioration in cell-mediated immunity as well as a broad host of other alterations in immune function that lead to the opportunistic infections and malignancies that characterize the clinical syndrome of the acquired immunodeficiency syndrome (AIDS). Although patients with AIDS and infections with the so-called atypical mycobacteria (*Mycobacterium avium-intracellulare* or *Mycobacterium. avium* complex) were noted early in the AIDS epidemic, it was not until recently that *Mycobacterium tuberculosis* was reported to be significantly associated with HIV infection and AIDS. Indeed, mycobacterial infections are the most frequent bacterial infections reported in AIDS. Since many patients with HIV infection are also in groups with a high prevalence of infection with *M tuberculosis* and are at risk for active disease as they develop immunosuppression, this represents an area of great public health concern. Other nontuberculous mycobacterial infections have also been diagnosed in patients with HIV infection and will be discussed briefly.

MYCOBACTERIUM TUBERCULOSIS INFECTION

Epidemiology

For 3 decades prior to 1985, the number of tuberculosis cases had decreased at a rate of 5–6% per year.[1,2] This rate of decline slowed significantly in 1985 and there was actually a slight increase in the number of cases in 1986.[2] This

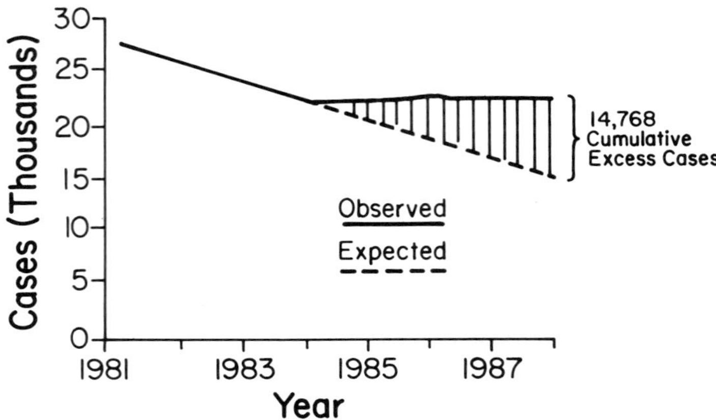

FIG. 1   Observed and expected tuberculosis cases in the United States, 1981–1988.

Independent risk factors for extrapulmonary tuberculosis among AIDS patients include black race, IV drug use, heterosexual AIDS transmission, and Hispanic ethnicity.

trend has continued through 1988, resulting in 14,768 more cases since 1984 than would have been predicted if the previous rates of decline had continued (Fig. 1).[1]

Even early in 1986, this lack of a continued decline in tuberculosis morbidity was postulated to be related to increases in tuberculosis cases among persons with HIV infection.[3] The earliest reports of tuberculosis in AIDS patients were from Florida where, from 1981 to 1985, 10% of reported AIDS cases had a diagnosis of tuberculosis.[4] Subsequently, reports from others areas with large numbers of AIDS cases also noted increasing tuberculosis morbidity.[5,6]

In the first reports of AIDS in Haitians from Miami it was noted that 50–60% of the patients had culture-proven tuberculosis.[7,8] Data from New York City from 1981 to 1985 revealed that overall, 5% of AIDS patients had a diagnosis of tuberculosis.[5] Hospital-based studies at two New York City hospitals showed rates of 7.8% and 8.6% for tuberculosis in patients with AIDS.[9,10] Whereas the reports from Miami had primarily noted tuberculosis in Haitian AIDS patients, these reports emphasized the prevalence in non-Haitians and noted the association with parenteral drug use.[9,10]

A recent review from Centers for Disease Control (CDC) of all AIDS cases reported from October 1987 (after the addition of extrapulmonary tuberculosis as an AIDS-defining condition)[11] through March 1989 revealed that 1,239 (2.5%) of 48,712 AIDS cases were diagnosed with extrapulmonary tuberculosis.[12] This likely represents an underestimate of the total number of AIDS patients with extrapulmonary tuberculosis since reporting of multiple diseases in the same person with AIDS is not mandatory and patients with extrapulmonary tuberculosis have had a prior or concomitant AIDS-defining condition in up to 50% of reported cases.[6,9,10] Extrapulmonary tuberculosis was diagnosed in 8% of Mexican-born and 13% of Haitian-born persons compared to 2.3% of U.S.-born persons with AIDS.[12] Independent risk factors for extrapulmonary tuberculosis among AIDS patients included black race, intravenous (IV) drug use, heterosexual AIDS transmission, and Hispanic ethnicity.[12]

A San Francisco study reviewed all cases of tuberculosis reported to the department of health from 1981 to 1985 and found that 12% of cases of tuberculosis in non-Asian-born men were in persons with AIDS.[11] Those with AIDS and tuberculosis were more likely to have a history of IV drug use than those with AIDS without tuberculosis.[11]

Other population groups with a high prevalence of tuberculosis infection and HIV infection, such as the homeless, are also at risk for increased tuberculosis morbidity.[13] A recent study of homeless men in a New York City shelter revealed that 67% of homeless men tested had a positive PPD reaction of 10 mm or greater with no difference between the HIV seropositive and HIV seronegative groups.[14] However, 27 (90%) of the 30 men with active tuberculous infection were HIV seropositive.[14]

Studies prior to 1985 were primarily the result of matching AIDS and tuberculosis registries and, therefore, could not address the prevalence of asymptomatic HIV infection among patients with tuberculosis. Two recent prospective studies from public health department clinics looked at the prevalence of seropositivity in patients newly diagnosed with tuberculosis and found that 22 (31%) of 71 consecutive patients with tuberculosis were HIV-seropositive in Miami[15] and 17 (28%) of 60 adult non-Asian-born patients with tuberculosis in San Francisco were seropositive for HIV.[16] Demographic characteristics of patients with tuberculosis who were HIV-seropositive from these two studies showed that they were more likely to be young adults (age range, 18–40 or 25–44 years), male, black, or Haitian. In addition, they were more likely to have a known risk factor for HIV infection, although 24% of patients from San Francisco who were seropositive denied any risk factors.[13,14] A blinded serosurvey of patients followed in the Boston City Tuberculosis Clinic showed a similar prevalence, with 26% of patients testing positive for HIV infection.[17]

Two recent prospective studies from public health department clinics found that the prevalence of HIV seropositivity in patients newly diagnosed with tuberculosis was 31% in Miami and 28% in San Francisco.

The risk of development of active tuberculous infection in HIV-seropositive individuals was further evaluated by Selwyn et al. in a prospective study of 519 IV drug users in a methadone-maintenance program in New York City.[18] Again, the prevalence of tuberculosis infection as measured by PPD reactivity was not significantly different between the two groups, with 23% of HIV-seropositive subjects and 20% of HIV-seronegative subjects having a positive PPD at baseline. However, over the 2-year period of the study, active tuberculosis developed in 8 of 215 HIV-seropositive subjects (4%) and none of the HIV-seronegative subjects ($P < .002$).

Tuberculosis in patients with HIV infection is not only a problem in the United States, but is of particular concern to many developing countries where it is one of the most common opportunistic infections in patients seropositive for HIV infection.[19] As many as 60% of tuberculosis patients are seropositive for HIV in central and east African countries.[19,20] Since many developing countries have a high rate of endemic tuberculosis infection, there is the potential for astronomical increases in tuberculosis morbidity in these areas if the same patients become immunocompromised due to HIV infection.[21] Even in Europe there has been a significant association of AIDS and tuberculosis, with reports of a tuberculosis diagnosis in 13 (6%) of 207 patients with AIDS from a London hospital and 67 (67%) of 100 patients with AIDS at a hospital in Madrid, Spain.[22,23]

Pathophysiology

Although *M tuberculosis* is generally regarded as an organism capable of causing disease in the normal host, an impairment in the cell-mediated immune response is the common predisposing factor for increased risk of active tuberculosis infection seen in a variety of conditions, as discussed in the chapter on pulmonary tuberculosis.

HIV infection causes both a quantitative and qualitative defect in the CD-4 (T-helper) lymphocyte population that is progressive over time.[24] In addition, macrophage function is diminished not only because of direct HIV infection, but also because there is a reduction in the elaboration of gamma interferon and interleukin-2 (IL-2) by HIV-infected T lymphocytes.[25] Thus, it is not surprising that initial infection with *M tuberculosis* would not be easily contained in the patient with HIV infection and significant immunosuppression, since containment is dependent upon the development of activated lymphocytes and macrophages.[26]

Although progressive primary tuberculosis infection would therefore be easily explained in patients with HIV infection, epidemiologic evidence suggests that tuberculosis infection in patients with HIV infection generally represents reactivation disease rather than progressive primary disease.[4,5,8] The reported AIDS patients with tuberculosis have been primarily Haitians, blacks, and Hispanics—groups known to have an increased endemic rate of tuberculosis infection. Also, the diagnosis of active tuberculosis for most AIDS/tuberculosis patients occurred clustered around the time of the AIDS diagnosis. More compelling evidence, moreover, comes from the Selwyn study in New York City in which seven of the eight HIV-seropositive subjects who developed active tuberculosis had a prior positive PPD, and the remaining subject had been previously anergic.[18] Although this is strong evidence for reactivation disease, the potential for primary disease is also noted, in that 15 (11%) of 131 HIV-seropositive and 26 (13%) of 202 seronegative IV drug abusers in this study converted from negative to positive PPD status over the 22-month follow-up period.[18]

Epidemiologic evidence suggests that tuberculosis infection in patients with HIV infection generally represents reactivation disease rather than progressive primary disease.

Clinical Manifestations

As might be expected, the clinical manifestations of tuberculosis in patients with HIV infection vary depending upon the degree of immunosuppression present at the time of diagnosis.[16,27] Since most published series have dealt primarily with patients who have clinical AIDS rather than asymptomatic HIV infection, there has been an emphasis on the atypical nature of tuberculosis with extrapulmonary disease, skin-test anergy, and diffuse pulmonary infiltrates.[6,8–9,10,13]

The clinical manifestations of tuberculosis in patients with HIV infection vary depending upon the degree of immunosuppression present at the time of diagnosis.

However, the series of adult non-Asian-born patients with tuberculosis from San Francisco showed no significant differences between the HIV seropositive and seronegative patients in terms of site of disease, skin-test reactivity, or response to therapy.[16] Tuberculosis was the first opportunistic infection in these patients, and only 2 of 17 had any clinical evidence of HIV infection prior to the diagnosis of tuberculosis. The mean $CD4^+$ lymphocyte count was $326/mm^3$ and was significantly lower ($CD4^+$ of 153) in those patients with extrapulmonary tuberculosis as compared to patients with pulmonary disease alone ($CD4^+$ of 367). Twelve (80%) of 15 HIV-positive patients tested had a tuberculin skin test with >10 mm induration compared to 27 (93%) of 29 HIV-seronegative patients. The three patients who had negative tuberculin skin tests all had extrapulmonary disease establishing the diagnosis of AIDS.[11] Pulmonary disease alone was seen in 13 (76%) of 17 HIV-positive patients compared to 31 (72%) of HIV-seronegative patients. No significant differences in the chest radiographic findings at the time of diagnosis were noted between the HIV seropositive and seronegative patients, as approximately half of all patients had focal infiltrates and a third had cavitary disease.[16]

An earlier HIV-seroprevalence study in tuberculosis patients from Miami found a somewhat more atypical disease presentation, but only 14 (64%) of the 22 HIV-seropositive tuberculosis patients had no clinical evidence of AIDS or AIDS-related complex (ARC) during the study period, implying a more significantly immunocompromised patient population.[15] CD4$^+$ lymphocyte counts are not given, making a direct comparison difficult, but only 9 (50%) of 18 HIV-seropositive subjects tested had a tuberculin skin test >10 mm, whereas 30 (91%) of 33 seronegative subjects tested had >10 mm induration (33% of seronegative subjects did not have skin tests placed). Pulmonary disease alone was diagnosed in 12 (55%) of 22 HIV-seropositive patients compared to 43 (88%) of 49 HIV-seronegative patients.

Studies in patients more extensively immunocompromised have shown that 50–72% of patients present with extrapulmonary disease.[6,8–10,13] Since extrapulmonary tuberculosis is now included as an AIDS-defining condition, these patients would now be considered to have AIDS.[11] In those series that have included reports of CD4$^+$ lymphocyte counts and have had a predominance of extrapulmonary disease,[8,17,21,28,29] mean CD4$^+$ lymphocyte counts have been significantly lower (range, 74–174) than in the series with more typical pulmonary involvement.[16] Lymph nodes were the most frequent site of extrapulmonary involvement seen in 27–33% of patients with tuberculosis and HIV infection. Other common sites include blood in 11–16%, urinary tract in 5–14%, bone marrow in 0–11%, gastrointestinal tract in 5–13%, pleura in 0–20%, musculoskeletal system in 0–9%, and soft tissue in 3–5%.[9,13,15,29] Unusual sites of involvement include the pancreas,[30] esophagus,[31] pericardium,[6] eye,[32] vertebrae[33,34] and skin.[35] Although one early series noted 3 (10.3%) of 29 patients with central nervous system (CNS) involvement,[6] subsequent reports have not confirmed such a high percentage.[36] Of the 10 subsequently reported patients with AIDS and CNS tuberculosis from the same New Jersey hospital as the earlier series, 8 had CNS mass lesions, whereas 2 presented with a picture of meningitis.[37] Nine of these 10 patients were intravenous drug abusers, two

Studies in patients more extensively immunocompromised have shown that 50–72% of patients present with extrapulmonary disease.

TABLE 1   Physical Findings in Patients With Concomitant HIV Infection and Tuberculosis

Mean temperature	39.2°C
Cachexia	40%
Tachypnea	36%
Oral thrush	37%
Generalized lymphadenopathy	31%
Localized lymphadenopathy	19%
Hepatomegaly	17%

of whom developed brain lesions while on therapy for extrapulmonary tuberculosis.

Symptoms of tuberculosis in patients with HIV infection are nonspecific and difficult to distinguish from symptoms attributable to HIV infection itself.[15,27] Fever and night sweats occur in 80–90% of patients, weight loss in 77–80%, and cough in 70–84%.[28,29] Physical findings are also nonspecific, as noted in Table 1.[28,29]

Chest roentgenographic (CXR) findings, as noted, were not significantly different in patients with asymptomatic HIV infection and tuberculosis and patients with tuberculosis who were HIV-seronegative.[16] Even in the modern pre-AIDS era, the "typical" CXR findings of upper lobe infiltrates with or without cavitation were *not* present in 34% of newly diagnosed pulmonary tuberculosis patients in Boston.[38] However, in patients who present with tuberculosis after or around the time of their AIDS diagnosis, upper lobe disease and cavitation are noted infrequently.[13,28,39] Hilar or mediastinal adenopathy is present in 20–59%, miliary or diffuse interstitial infiltrates in 15–60%, pleural effusions in 12–28%, cavitation of 0–18%, and no abnormality noted in 6–40%.[6,13,15,28,29,39,40]

The ability to mount a delayed hypersensitivity reaction is impaired in advanced HIV disease and is reflected in the reported low frequency of positive tuberculin skin-test reactions in patients with HIV infection and active tuberculosis, with a range of 7–50% noted to have reactions >9 mm.[7,10,13,15,28] However, in the prospective study by Theuer et al., which included mostly asymptomatic HIV-seropositive patients with tuberculosis, 80% with active tuberculosis had positive reactions.[16]

Diagnosis

The definitive diagnosis of tuberculosis in patients with HIV infection depends upon isolation of the organism from clinical specimens. Although the presence of acid-fast ba-

Chest roentgenographic findings were not significantly different in patients with asymptomatic HIV infection and tuberculosis and patients with tuberculosis who were HIV-seronegative.

Since the signs and symptoms of tuberculosis in HIV-seropositive patients are nonspecific, a high index of suspicion must be held as diagnostic evaluation is undertaken.

cilli (AFB) in such specimens is indicative of mycobacterial disease, atypical mycobacteria are also a common cause of disease in this patient population and can be distinguished definitively only by identification of the organism from culture material.[41] Although there has long been interest in the development of serologic tests for mycobacterial infection, rapid immunodiagnostic techniques based on the detection of either mycobacterial antigens or antibodies have not become available for widespread clinical use, as has been the case for other infectious diseases, such as fungal infections.[42,43] Since the signs and symptoms of tuberculosis in HIV-seropositive patients are nonspecific, as previously noted, a high index of suspicion must be held as diagnostic evaluation is undertaken.

Although CXR findings are variable depending upon the stage of HIV infection, hilar adenopathy on CXR is not associated with *Pneumocystic carinii* pneumonia and should raise a strong suspicion of mycobacterial disease or malignancy.[44] Most series show no significant difference between HIV-seropositive and seronegative subjects with tuberculosis in regard to the frequency of AFB positive sputum smears.[15,16,29] However, one report from New York found that only 45% of AIDS/ARC patients with culture-positive pulmonary tuberculosis had a positive AFB smear compared to 81% in a nonAIDS/ARC control group with the initial sputum smear positive in only 29%.[45] The presence of either granulomas or acid-fast organisms in bronchoscopic material suggests the possibility of tuberculosis and allows for empiric therapy while awaiting the results of mycobacterial cultures.

In patients with any clinical or laboratory evidence of possible extrapulmonary disease, the site involved should be evaluated by acid-fast smear and culture of biopsy or aspiration material. Sites that should be considered include lymph nodes, bone marrow, liver, urine, spinal fluid, pleural fluid, stool, blood, and other tissues or fluids as clinically indicated.[28,29,41,46,47] In a study from New York, 12 (46%) of 27 patients with generalized lymphadenopathy who underwent lymph node biopsy for evaluation of AIDS had a positive culture for tuberculosis.[48] Histologic examination showed granulomas in eight (30%) with caseation in seven.[48] However, since the classic histologic findings of caseating granulomas occur less frequently in patients with AIDS and tuberculosis, the absence of granulomas does not rule out tuberculosis, and all specimens should be cultured for mycobacteria and have specific stains for acid-fast organisms.[10,47]

M tuberculosis bacteremia in an AIDS patient was first reported in an IV drug abuser from New York utilizing a

> *Since the classic histologic findings of caseating granulomas occur less frequently in patients with AIDS and tuberculosis, the absence of granulomas does not rule out tuberculosis, and all specimens should be cultured for mycobacteria and have specific stains for acid-fast organisms.*

radiometric blood culture system.[49] Since then, 26–64% of selected patients with tuberculosis and HIV infection have been shown to have positive blood cultures by a variety of methods, but most commonly the BACTEC radiometric system and the DuPont Isolator lysis-centrifugation system.[17,23,28,29,50,51] The mean time to detection of a positive blood culture for *M tuberculosis* was 40–44 days (range, 20–75 days)[17,47,50] Identification of the isolates as *M tuberculosis* can be accomplished within hours by use of nucleic acid probes if isolated colonies are available.[52] However, some laboratories either do not use this expensive technique, or hold the culture and run the probes in batches rather than individually, thereby delaying a definitive identification.[17] Although the majority of patients with blood cultures positive for *M tuberculosis* have positive cultures from other sites or have died prior to the blood culture becoming positive,[17,50] combinations of new methods that attempt to provide a more rapid diagnosis may make blood culturing for mycobacteria a more clinically useful diagnostic technique.[52]

A recent review of all HIV-infected patients with tuberculosis seen at a Los Angeles medical center over a 7-month period sought to determine the frequency of a delayed diagnosis of tuberculosis and the reasons for such delays.[28] In 25 of 52 patients, tuberculosis was untreated prior to the patients' death or treated more than 22 days after presentation for evaluation. Delayed diagnosis was not due to atypical manifestations of tuberculosis, but rather to failure to consider the diagnosis and obtain appropriate clinical specimens for acid-fast smear and culture (such as three sputum specimens in patients with respiratory symptoms and/or an abnormal chest radiograph or obtaining a bone marrow examination in a patient with marked anemia).[28]

Delayed diagnosis of tuberculosis was not due to atypical manifestations, but rather to failure to consider the diagnosis and obtain appropriate clinical specimens for acid-fast smear and culture.

Treatment

Most *M tuberculosis* isolates from HIV-infected patients are susceptible to first-line antituberculous agents.[6,10] The recommended regimen for adult HIV-infected patients with tuberculosis includes isoniazid (INH), plus rifampin, plus pyrazinamide, with ethambutol added if CNS or disseminated disease is present or INH resistance is suspected, as noted in Table 2.[46]

Drug susceptibility tests should be done on all isolates, with revision of the regimen if resistance is noted to any of the prescribed drugs. The optimal duration of therapy for patients with HIV infection and tuberculosis is not known. However, the CDC and American Thoracic Society recommend that treatment be given for a minimum of 9

TABLE 2   Recommended Regimen for HIV-Seropositive Adults With Tuberculosis

Drug	Dosage
Isoniazid	300 mg/day
Rifampin	600 mg/day or 450 mg if <50 kg
Pyrazanimide	20–30 mg/kg/day during first 2 months of therapy
Ethambutol*	25 mg/kg/day

* Should be included when central nervous system or disseminated disease is present or isoniazid (INH) resistance is suspected until susceptibility tests are available.

Clinical experience in treating HIV-seropositive patients with tuberculosis with standard chemotherapeutic agents has been generally quite favorable, with rapid resolution of symptoms and radiographic abnormalities.

months, with at least 6 months of therapy after the last documented positive culture.[46] Some authorities suggest lifelong INH therapy because of the potential for relapse in these immunocompromised patients,[53] analogous to the lifelong maintenance therapy given for most other opportunistic infections in patients with AIDS. If either INH or rifampin is not included in the regimen, therapy should be continued for a minimum of 18 months.

Clinical experience in treating HIV-seropositive patients with tuberculosis with standard chemotherapeutic agents has been generally quite favorable, with rapid resolution of symptoms and radiographic abnormalities.[54] No difference in time-to-sputum conversion from positive to negative has been observed between HIV-seropositive and seronegative patients.[10,15,16] Small et al., in a recent retrospective analysis of the outcomes in 132 patients with both AIDS and tuberculosis from San Francisco, noted no relapses in patients who completed a standard course of therapy and were compliant.[54] Although at least 20 months had elapsed since the diagnosis of tuberculosis for all 125 of the treated patients, median survival of these patients was only 16 months from the time of diagnosis.[54] Follow-up periods in these studies, however, have been short, with an average period of 9.5–10 months after completion of therapy.[10,16,54] Sunderham et al. reported three apparent treatment failures, two of whom had progressive CNS involvement, and one who had pericardial disease, despite receiving appropriate therapy.[6] This provides further support for the recommendation that patients be followed closely for the rest of their lives with evaluation for relapse if clinical symptoms or signs are noted.[27,46] Patients with a history of noncompliance should be considered for supervised, directly administered therapy.[46]

Early studies suggested an increased incidence of adverse drug reactions to antituberculous drugs in patients with HIV infection.[13] Two recent series of HIV-infected patients with tuberculosis have not shown a significant difference in toxicity between HIV-seropositive and seronegative patients.[15,16] However, in patients with tuberculosis and the diagnosis of AIDS (not just HIV-seropositive) from San Francisco, there was a significant increase in adverse drug reactions, especially to rifampin.[10,54] In Africa, significant increases in cutaneous hypersensitivity reactions, including Stevens-Johnson syndrome, have been seen in patients treated with regimens containing thiacetazone.[19,20]

It is important to remember that antituberculous chemotherapy should be initiated whenever acid-fast bacilli are seen on a smear from clinical material in a patient with HIV infection until the organism is definitively identified.[46] Many would also suggest that antituberculous therapy be initiated in a patient with symptoms or signs compatible with the diagnosis of tuberculosis while awaiting the results of cultures of appropriate clinical specimens if no other etiology for the abnormalities has been found.[28] Kramer et al. noted that 85% of their HIV-infected patients with tuberculosis defervesced during the first week of therapy; they suggest that a therapeutic trial of antituberculous therapy may be diagnostically useful in this setting.[28]

Antituberculous chemotherapy should be initiated whenever acid-fast bacilli are seen on a smear from clinical material in a patient with HIV infection until the organism is definitively identified.

Prevention and Infection Control

Since HIV-seropositive patients with tuberculosis infection are at significant risk of active tuberculous disease as their immune system deteriorates,[15] *all* HIV-infected patients should have tuberculin skin testing performed when they are first noted to be HIV-seropositive.[55] The current recommendation is that all HIV-seropositive individuals with ≥5 mm of induration to 5 TU of purified protein derivative (PPD) be considered to have tuberculous infection.[55] A chest radiograph should be done to evaluate the patient for active disease, and sputum samples should be obtained for acid-fast stain and culture if the CXR is abnormal or if the patient has respiratory symptoms.[46] After active disease is ruled out, all HIV-seropositive patients with a positive skin test should then be given INH 300 mg daily for 12 months, regardless of age or history of prior positive test.[55] There is now some data to suggest that INH prophylaxis is effective in prevention of active tuberculosis in HIV-infected patients. Selwyn et al. noted that among HIV-seropositive patients with a prior positive PPD test no cases of active tuberculosis developed in subjects who had received INH prophylaxis.[18] Although this difference was not statistically significant, it suggests that prophylaxis may be efficacious in this population.[18] A prospective pla-

All HIV-infected patients should have tuberculin skin testing performed when they are first noted to be HIV-seropositive.

cebo-controlled study from Zambia in patients with HIV-infection showed that INH prophylaxis significantly reduced the incidence of active *M tuberculosis* infection.[56] None of 190 patients treated with INH for 6 months developed active tuberculosis, whereas 5 (4.4%) of 220 patients who received placebo developed active disease with follow-up periods of 99 and 113 patient years, respectively.[56]

Because of reports of local reactions and disseminated disease after the administration of bacille Calmette-Guérin (BCG) vaccination in HIV-infected patients, BCG should not be given to symptomatic HIV-infected persons.[57] Its use should be reserved for asymptomatic HIV-infected persons in geographic areas where tuberculosis is highly endemic and the potential risks for disseminated disease are outweighed by the risk of active tuberculosis. BCG does not have a role in prevention of *M tuberculosis* infection in the United States and other developed countries at this time.

Tuberculosis is the only HIV-related infection that is transmissible from person to person, including other HIV-infected persons and health care workers.

Tuberculosis is the only HIV-related infection that is transmissible from person to person, including other HIV-infected persons and health-care workers. Recent reports of nosocomial transmission of *M tuberculosis* infection from patients with HIV infection have shown that this is more than a theoretical concern.[58–60] In a Florida clinic, transmission of tuberculosis was epidemiologically linked to administration of aerosolized pentamidine in a poorly ventilated setting.[59] An outbreak in Italy that resulted in active tuberculosis in eight HIV-infected patients and one health care worker was traced to an index patient who had fever and cough but a normal chest radiograph and, therefore, remained undiagnosed for 28 days, until cultures from a bronchoscopy were positive for *M tuberculosis*.[58] This emphasizes the need to utilize respiratory isolation for all HIV-infected patients with pulmonary symptoms until tuberculosis can be ruled out.

Since pulmonary tuberculosis can present in an atypical fashion in patients with HIV infection, one must strongly consider tuberculosis in the diagnosis of any HIV-seropositive patient with fever and respiratory symptoms, even in those patients with a normal chest radiograph.

More recently, documented nosocomial transmission of multidrug-resistant tuberculosis occurred among HIV-infected patients and health-care workers in a Florida hospital in which failure to follow all recommendations for respiratory isolation was implicated as a contributing factor in the outbreak.[60] Currently it is recommended that patients with suspected or confirmed tuberculosis remain in respiratory isolation until clinically improved, with a decrease in number of organisms on sputum smears and a reduction in cough.[60] Sputum induction and aerosolized pentamidine treatments should ideally be administered in single-patient rooms or booths that have negative air pressure in relation to adjacent rooms or hallways and should be exhausted directly outside.[59] In geographic areas with significant drug-resistant *M tuberculosis* infection, patients should remain in respiratory isolation until acid-fast smears are negative, since drug-susceptibility tests often take weeks to months to become available. Since pulmonary tuberculosis can present in an atypical fashion in patients with HIV infection, one must strongly consider tuberculosis in the diagnosis of any HIV-seropositive patient with fever and respiratory symptoms, even in those patients with normal chest radiograph.[39] To miss the diagnosis not only denies the patient therapy for a treatable infection, but also puts health-care workers and other patients and family members at risk for acquiring tuberculous infection.

MYCOBACTERIUM AVIUM COMPLEX INFECTION

Mycobacterium avium and *Mycobacterium intracellulare* are two closely related nontuberculous mycobacteria often grouped together as the *Mycobacterium avium-intracellulare* complex (MAC).[61] They are nonchromogenic, Runyon group III organisms that, prior to the AIDS epidemic, primarily caused progressive pulmonary infection in patients with underlying lung disease.[61] Disseminated infection occurred in only 37 patients reviewed from 1940 to 1984 who did not have AIDS; however, most had some preexisting condition associated with altered immunity.[62] Since 1981, disseminated infection with MAC has been frequently identified in patients with AIDS[63,64] and has been one of the most difficult opportunistic infections to treat in these patients.[65,66] Indeed, there is still a great deal of debate regarding when and whether to initiate therapy and the optimal regimen to employ in treating MAC infection in patients with AIDS.[66–68]

Epidemiology

From June 1981 through August 1987, 2,269 cases of disseminated nontuberculous mycobacterial infections were reported to the CDC in patients with AIDS, of which 96% were due to *M avium* complex.[69] Patients with disseminated nontuberculous mycobacterial infection represented 5.5% of AIDS cases reported over the same time period. In retrospective series, 17–34% of AIDS patients have been diagnosed with MAC infection during life.[70–74] Autopsy

*Unlike infection due to **M tuberculosis**, MAC infection occurs primarily in patients with severe compromise of the immune system.*

series, however, reveal evidence of disseminated disease in 40–53% of AIDS patients.[71,75] Of 50 patients at Sloan-Kettering Cancer Center diagnosed with MAC infection before death, 48 had already been diagnosed with an AIDS-defining condition 1–24 (mean, 9.3) months prior to the diagnosis of MAC infection.[71] In a series from Los Angeles, all of the 55 patients with MAC infection had a preexisting diagnosis of AIDS. This is in contrast to HIV-seropositive patients with tuberculosis in whom the diagnosis of AIDS preceded the diagnosis of tuberculosis in only 13 (33%) of 39 cases.[29] Indeed, in an Atlanta study, 14 (36%) of 39 HIV-seropositive patients with $CD4^+$ lymphocyte counts below 100 had positive blood cultures for MAC, whereas none of 41 with $CD4^+$ lymphocytes of >100 had positive blood cultures.[76] This data suggests that, unlike infection due to *M tuberculosis*, MAC infection occurs primarily in patients with severe compromise of the immune system.

Disseminated MAC was less common in AIDS cases with Kaposi sarcoma and Hispanics and declined with age.[69] Otherwise, no significant differences were shown in patient sex or mode of transmission of HIV infection between AIDS patients with and without reported MAC infection.[69] This is in contrast to the data presented for *M tuberculosis* infection in which the majority of cases have been in patient groups with a high prevalence of tuberculous infection, such as Haitians, Hispanics, and IV drug abusers.[12]

Although MAC infection has been reported in a significant percentage of patients with AIDS in Australia,[73] London,[20] and Berlin,[77] reports from Africa have noted tuberculosis as the only significant mycobacterial infection in patients with HIV infection.[19] This lack of significant MAC infections in African HIV-infected patients is supported by a recent study from Uganda, in which none of 50 patients with advanced AIDS had a positive blood culture for MAC.[78]

M avium complex is a ubiquitous environmental organism that has been isolated from water, soil, dust, and a variety of domestic and wild animals.[79] Serotyping of MAC isolates from AIDS patients has shown that serotypes 4 and 8 of *M avium* are the most commonly encountered in the United States.[80] Genetic probes specific for *M avium* and *M intracellulare* have been used against isolates of MAC revealing that 98% of isolates from AIDS patients are *M avium*, whereas in non-AIDS patients with respiratory infection, 54% of the isolates are *M intracellulare*.[81] Whether the serotypes noted with increased frequency are actually more virulent or merely reflect a common source of exposure is not clear.

Pathophysiology

The epidemiologic data cited above suggest that *M avium* complex infection in HIV-seropositive patients represents newly acquired infection following colonization with organisms from the environment, rather than reactivation of latent infection, as in most cases of *M tuberculosis* infection. However, the initial portal of entry for *M avium* complex is still a matter of debate.[74] Ingestion of organisms in water or contaminated food, with subsequent entry through the gastrointestinal (GI) tract has been proposed by some on the basis of the observation that AIDS patients often have large numbers of organisms in the lower GI tract as well as clusters within macrophages in the wall of the small bowel.[71,74,82] Other data suggest that aerosolizaton and inhalation of the organism, followed by dissemination from the respiratory tract analagous to the pathogenesis of tuberculosis, is the likely mode of infection.[83] This theory is supported by Hawkins' series in which respiratory secretions were culture-positive for MAC in 30 (75%) of 40 patients who had respiratory cultures, whereas only 13 (36%) of 36 patients had positive stool cultures for MAC.[71] Since MAC is ubiquitous in the environment, it may be that infection can occur by either route.

Since *M avium* complex is an intracellular pathogen taken up by macrophages, the defects in cell-mediated immunity, which occur with HIV and are associated with increased susceptibility to active tuberculous infection, likely also play a major role in susceptibility to MAC infection. However, the precise mechanisms of host response to MAC infection are not well delineated, although some evidence suggests that natural killer (NK) cell function is important in the control of MAC infection.[84] Additionally, a factor found in normal human serum that inhibits growth of *M avium* in human macrophages has been found to be lacking in the sera of some AIDS patients.[85] Thus, it is likely that a number of factors are responsible for the predilection of AIDS patients to acquire disseminated infection with MAC at the rate observed.

Clinical Manifestations

Since disseminated MAC infection occurs late in the course of AIDS, multiple infectious and malignant processes are often present concomitantly, making it difficult to delineate the signs and symptoms that are specific to MAC infection.[40,63,64,71] Indeed, some patients may have MAC isolated from blood, bone marrow, or stool at a time when

The epidemiologic data suggest that **M** *avium* **complex** *infection in HIV-seropositive patients represents newly acquired infection following colonization with organisms from the environment rather than reactivation of latent infection, as in most cases of* **M** **tuberculosis** *infection.*

they are relatively asymptomatic with only occasional low-grade fevers.[74] In non-AIDS patients with disseminated MAC, the most common symptoms included fever, weight loss, and localized pain.[62] Similar symptoms have also been noted frequently in AIDS patients with disseminated MAC infection.[22,29,40,71,86] Hawkins et al. reported fever, malaise, and weight loss occurring in almost every patient who was considered to have infection with MAC.[71] These symptoms preceded the diagnosis of MAC infection by several months. In other series of patients with AIDS and MAC infection, cough and diarrhea were more frequently reported than in the series of non-AIDS patients with disseminated MAC, as noted in Table 3.[22,29,40,62,86]

Physical findings in AIDS patients with MAC infection are also nonspecific but commonly include fever and cachexia.[29,71] Generalized lymphadenopathy, hepatomegaly, or splenomegaly have been reported in patients with disseminated MAC infection, but are also seen in other opportunistic infections and malignancies associated with AIDS.[22,29,65] Normochromic, normocytic anemia is the most common laboratory finding, with a mean hemoglobin level of 8.6–8.9 g/dL.[29,63,86] Liver enzymes are also commonly elevated, but no specific pattern has been noted.[40,63]

Gastrointestinal involvement has been reported frequently in AIDS patients with disseminated MAC infection manifested by mild to severe abdominal pain, diarrhea, and malabsorption.[22,29,65,71,86] In Hawkins' series, chronic diarrhea and abdominal pain were prominent symptoms in 11 patients who subsequently were shown to have MAC infection of bowel by biopsy or autopsy findings.[71] In a series of 81 HIV-seropositive patients from London with persistent noncryptosporidial diarrhea, 10 (12%) were

> *Gastrointestinal involvement has been reported frequently in AIDS patients with disseminated MAC infection manifested by mild to severe abdominal pain, diarrhea, and malabsorption.*

TABLE 3   Symptoms Reported in Patients With Disseminated MAC

	Non-AIDS		AIDS	
	Patients	%	Patients	%
Fever	20/37	54	44/50	88
Weight loss	12/37	32	*	*
Cough	8/37	22	36/51	70
Local pain	12/37	32		
Chest	3/37	8		
Abdominal	16/43	37		
Diarrhea	3/37	8	32/51	63

* patients had a mean weight loss of 10.5 kg
MAC, *Mycobacterium avium-intracellulare complex*; AIDS, acquired immune deficiency syndrome
Data from references 33 and 68.

found to have MAC infection of the GI tract.[87] MAC was the pathogen most frequently isolated in this study, and was associated with weight loss of more than 10 kg and hemoglobin of less than 10 g/dL. Others have reported small bowel involvement with MAC, producing a clinical picture that resembles Whipple's disease with fever and malabsorption.[88,89] These patients have aggregates of foamy macrophages containing acid-fast bacteria in the lamina propria of the small bowel often associated with enlarged mesenteric lymph nodes with similar histologic findings.[71,8] In two reported patients with MAC infection, enlarged peripancreatic and portahepatic lymph nodes have been associated with the clinical picture of extrahepatic biliary tract obstruction with jaundice.[71] Terminal ileitis resembling Crohn's disease has also been described due to MAC infection in a patient with AIDS.[90]

Nonspecific respiratory symptoms, such as cough and shortness of breath, have been reported in approximately one-half of the HIV-infected patients with MAC.[22,29,40,91] However, many of these patients had concurrent pulmonary processes that may have contributed to their respiratory symptoms.[29,40,91] Chest radiographic findings are nonspecific but include diffuse interstitial infiltrates in approximately 50%, hilar or mediastinal adenopathy in 11–20%, alveolar infiltrates in 20%, and a normal chest radiograph in 14–22%.[29,40,91,92] Cavitary disease and pleural effusions are distinctly unusual in these patients.[29,40,71,91]

In contrast to pulmonary tuberculosis in HIV-seropositive patients, pulmonary MAC infection has generally been part of a disseminated infection.[29] However, two AIDS patients were recently described with endobronchial lesions due to MAC infection, causing obstruction and hilar adenopathy suggestive of a malignancy, but with negative blood and urine cultures for MAC.[93] Both of these patients were on zidovudine, and the authors suggest that the vigorous inflammatory response noted pathologically and the localization of infection might be a result of partial restoration of the immune response to MAC infection due to zidovudine. These patients did well with endoscopic debridement of the lesions and antimycobacterial therapy.

In contrast to pulmonary tuberculosis in HIV-seropositive patients, pulmonary MAC infection has generally been part of a disseminated infection.

Barbaro has also suggested an alteration in the natural history of MAC infection in patients on zidovudine therapy in his report of three patients with AIDS and localized cutaneous abscesses in lymphatic areas caused by MAC, with negative cultures of blood and bone marrow and no symptoms of disseminated infection.[94] All three patients were treated with incision and drainage as well as a short course of antimycobacterial therapy and had healing of the lesions, although one patient went on to develop disseminated infection with MAC 8 months after the initial diagnosis and died 2 months later.[94]

Although *M avium* complex has been cultured from the brain of patients with AIDS at autopsy, the clinical significance of these findings is unclear, since most of the patients had known disseminated MAC infection and often had histologic evidence of other pathologic processes of the CNS.[36,95] Other unusual manifestations of MAC infection include endophthalmitis[96] and chronic pericarditis.[97]

Diagnosis

M avium complex has been isolated from a variety of clinical specimens from patients with HIV infection, including blood, bone marrow, respiratory secretions, stool, urine, and biopsy specimens of liver, lymph nodes, bowel, and spleen.[29,40,71,72,82,86,98] The diagnostic yield of mycobacterial cultures of various clinical specimens is outlined in Table 4.[29,71,86,98] Although current blood culture techniques, such as the Dupont Isolator lysis-centrifugation system or the BACTEC radiometric system, have a very high yield in disseminated disease, there is still a delay in diagnosis while awaiting growth and identification of the organism.[52,98–100] A rough correlation was noted between the number of colonies and the time to positive culture, but no significant difference was seen between the two methods in percent of recovery of mycobacteria. The average time to detection of a positive culture was 14–24 days (range, 7–57 days).[52,99,100]

TABLE 4   Frequency of Positive Antemortem Cultures for MAC From Various Clinical Specimens

	Hawkins[77] n (%)	Modilevsky[33] n (%)	Wallace[93] n (%)
Blood	45/46 (98)	47/49 (96)	18/21 (86)
Bone marrow	14/14 (100)	10/17 (59)	2/5 (40)
Liver	6/6 (100)	ND	ND
Sputum	16/22 (73)	23/25 (92)	11/38 (29)
Bronchoscopic specimen	14/18 (78)	7/17 (41)	6/23 (26)
Lymph node	3/3 (100)	1/2 (50)	ND
Stool	13/36 (36)	15/20 (75)	3/5 (60)
Urine	12/28 (43)	ND	1/3 (33)

Data from references 33, 77, and 93
ND, not done

Patients with AIDS have been reported to have continuous high-grade MAC bacteremia, with colony counts of up to 28,000 colony-forming units (cfu)/mL.[98,101] In addition, buffy coat smears have been noted to show acid-fast bacilli in patients with MAC bacteremia.[102,103] Although one report found positive acid-fast stains of buffy coat smears in 13 of 14 patients with a positive blood culture for MAC,[102] a subsequent report found positive smears in only 6 (35%) of 17 patients who were mycobacteremic.[103] Even though the sensitivity is low, this is a rapid, simple procedure with 100% specificity for mycobacteremia and should be considered in conjunction with obtaining blood cultures in AIDS patients with unexplained fevers, progressive weight loss, and diarrhea.[68,103] Two blood cultures utilizing either the lysis-centrifugation or radiometric method specific for mycobacteria appear to be sufficient for the detection of mycobacteremia in AIDS patients.[104,105]

Patients with AIDS have been reported to have continuous high-grade bacteremia.

Two blood cultures utilizing either the lysis-centrifugation or radiometric method specific for mycobacteria appear to be sufficient for the detection of mycobacteremia in AIDS patients.

Although most AIDS patients with disseminated MAC infection eventually have positive blood cultures, smears and cultures of other clinical specimens may be positive earlier.[106] Bone marrow smears and cultures were the best indicators of early disseminated infection, with positive results preceding positive blood cultures by 4–5 weeks in some patients.[48,98,106] In a series of 51 bone marrow aspirates and biopsies from 47 patients with HIV infection, 18 (35.3%) were culture-positive for mycobacteria, and in 13 of 18, imprints from the biopsy samples were also positive for acid-fast bacilli by auramine-rhodamine fluorescent staining.[107] Although 10 of the 18 culture-positive samples in this series contained granulomas, other reports have emphasized the importance of routine acid-fast staining and culture for mycobacteria in all bone marrow specimens from AIDS patients since granulomas are frequently not seen.[47,107]

Liver biopsies have also been useful in more rapid diagnosis of disseminated MAC infection in symptomatic patients.[47] Indeed, in a series of liver biopsies in 26 AIDS patients, MAC infection was diagnosed in 8 (31%), 7 of whom had both granulomas and acid-fast organisms noted on histologic examination.[109] Prego found that histologic examination of liver biopsy tissue is the most rapid means of diagnosis of mycobacterial disease in HIV-infected patients with fever of undetermined origin.[47]

Histologic examination of liver biopsy tissue is the most rapid means of diagnosis of mycobacterial disease in HIV-infected patients with fever of undetermined origin.

Acid-fast stains and cultures of fecal specimens are a noninvasive and relatively rapid method of detecting the presence of mycobacteria, although they do not prove that disseminated disease is present.[71,82,98,106] Although Hawkins found that all 13 patients who had acid-fast bacilli noted on stool smears had positive stool cultures for MAC and evidence of disseminated infection,[71] other studies have reported that less than 50% of patients with positive stool cultures for MAC had documented disseminated disease.[106,110] However, the detection of mycobacteria in the stool may precede the detection of dissemination by other means by weeks to months.[74,106]

Although isolation of MAC from respiratory secretions may represent colonization in some patients,[92] disseminated disease with positive cultures from blood or other sterile sites is frequently detected with subsequent screening.[71,106] Bronchoscopic specimens from bronchoalveolar lavage or transbronchial biopsy should be cultured for mycobacteria even if acid-fast organisms are not seen on stains, since cultures have a significantly higher yield than smears alone.[45,111]

The histopathology of biopsy specimens from AIDS patients with disseminated MAC characteristically shows poorly formed granulomas with large numbers of acid-fast organisms in striated histiocytes or foamy macrophages.

The histopathology of biopsy specimens from AIDS patients with disseminated MAC characteristically shows poorly formed granulomas with large numbers of acid-fast organisms in striated histiocytes or foamy macrophages.[86,90,112] Features of typical granulomatous inflammation, such as Langhans giant cells, lymphocytic infiltrates, epithelioid histiocytes, fibrosis, and calcification, are rarely seen.[112] The presence of MAC infection is strongly suggested by the presence of numerous negatively staining rod-shaped spaces within histiocytes and in extracellular material on cytologic preparations from aspirated material from lymph nodes, bone marrow, or bronchoalveolar lavage specimens.[113,114] Thus, routine cytology may suggest the diagnosis even before special stains and cultures are available.

Although routine chest radiographs are nonspecific in patients with AIDS and MAC infection, gallium imaging may be useful in the evaluation of the symptomatic AIDS patient to suggest MAC infection.[115,116] In one series of gallium scans in symptomatic patients suspected of having AIDS, 9 of 10 scans with abnormal focal gallium uptake involving parahilar, mediastinal, supraclavicular, and/or cervical lymph node areas occurred in association with MAC infection.[116] Since lymphoma is also associated with nodal uptake by gallium, a suggestive gallium scan should be followed by needle aspiration or excisional biopsy of accessible lymph nodes. Retroperitoneal and mesenteric lymphadenopathy as demonstrated by abdominal computed tomography examination is also suggestive of MAC infection and should lead to further evaluation to confirm the diagnosis by cytology and culture.[117]

Therapy and Prognosis

No clear consensus exists regarding the optimal therapeutic regimen for the treatment of *M avium* complex infection in HIV-seropositive patients. Indeed, there is debate regarding whether disseminated MAC should be treated with specific antimycobacterial therapy or whether only palliative therapy should be given for symptom control.[66–68] It is not surprising that treatment of MAC infection in AIDS patients would be difficult. Not only is MAC relatively resistant to many antimycobacterial agents in vitro, but its intracellular location requires that agents be able to gain entry to and have activity within the macrophage.[68,118,119] Additionally, the marked immunosuppression of these patients would make bactericidal activity of any regimen an important component.[118]

Unfortunately, no standardized methods exist for the in vitro susceptibility testing of mycobacteria other than *M tuberculosis* making it difficult to assess the utility of in vitro testing.[119,120] Isolates have been uniformly resistant to isoniazid and pyrazinamide.[119] Occasional strains are susceptible to rifampin, but other rifamycins, including rifabutin and especially rifapentine, are generally more active in vitro.[121] Ethambutol, which is primarily tuberculostatic against *M tuberculosis*, is tuberculocidal against many MAC strains and has been shown to enhance the susceptibility of MAC to other antimycobacterial drugs, such as rifampin, ciprofloxacin, and ofloxacin, probably by inhibition of cell envelope synthesis.[122–123] Aminoglycosides, other than capreomycin, are some of the more active agents in vitro, with a slight advantage noted for amikacin in some studies.[125] Almost half of the tested strains were susceptible to clofazamine in one study, with all clinical strains considered susceptible in another report.[71,119]

Studies in the beige mouse model, an immunodeficient strain of mice with an increased susceptibility to MAC infection, have provided some in vivo data regarding agents and combinations of agents that may have activity, but the predictability of this information for outcome in human disease has yet to be proven.[68,126] The combination of amikacin or kanamycin and clofazamine appeared to be the most active combination of currently available drugs that were studied.[126,127]

Initial reports of therapy for MAC infection in humans were quite disappointing.[71,75] Hawkins, from Memorial Sloan-Kettering Cancer Center, treated 29 patients with various combinations, including ansamycin (rifabutin) and clofazamine, plus a variety of other drugs in most pa-

> *Not only is MAC relatively resistant to many antimycobacterial agents in vitro, but its intracellular location requires that agents be able to gain entry to and have activity within the macrophage.*

tients.[71] Despite in vitro data showing that the isolates were susceptible to ansamycin and clofazamine, all 29 patients had evidence of persistent MAC infection despite treatment. Only three patients had a reduction in colony counts of MAC in blood cultures, and there were no significant improvements in symptoms thought secondary to MAC infection. Similar findings were reported by Masur in 13 patients with persistent mycobacteremia treated with clofazamine and ansamycin, with amikacin or other drugs added in some patients based upon in vitro susceptibilities.[75] Although six patients had two or more negative blood cultures at some time during therapy, in only one patient did a clinical correlation exist between resolution of symptoms and conversion of blood culture to negative.

Somewhat more promising data was presented by Baron, who treated four patients with amikacin, ethambutol, and rifampin after in vitro studies suggested synergistic activity of these three agents against the patients' isolates.[128] All four patients had clinical improvement with clearing of mycobacteremia in the three patients with follow-up blood cultures; however, all three patients subsequently died.

Agins treated seven patients with disseminated MAC infection and three patients with positive cultures only from the respiratory tract with a combination of ansamycin (rifabutin) 150 mg/day, clofazamine, ethambutol, and isoniazid.[129] Six of seven patients with disseminated disease had improvement in clinical symptoms and cleared their bacteremia, but only one lived for more than a year after the onset of mycobacteremia. These encouraging results were substantiated by the Hoy series from Australia, in which mycobacteremia was cleared in 22 of 25 patients who received essentially the same regimen except that the dose of rifabutin was higher at 300–600 mg/day.[73] Eighteen of these 22 patients had complete resolution of symptoms associated with MAC infection, but bacteremia recurred in 6 patients over time, and 3 of 6 patients who had autopsies had positive cultures for MAC.

A regimen including amikacin with ethambutol, rifampin, and ciprofloxacin was reported by the California Collaborative Treatment Group to show a reduced level of bacteremia in 15 of 17 patients who received at least 4 weeks of therapy associated with an improvement in symptoms.[130] Only 10 patients completed the planned 12 weeks of therapy; 3 had clearing of bacteremia, 5 had a reduction in colony-forming units, and 2 had increased bacteremia. Therapy was terminated early primarily because of gastrointestinal intolerance of the regimen or hepatic toxicity. Amikacin 7.5 mg/kg/day was given for only the first 4

Eighteen of 22 patients had complete resolution of symptoms associated with MAC infection, but bacteremia recurred in 6 patients over time, and 3 of 6 patients who had autopsies had positive cultures for MAC.

weeks of therapy, and no significant toxicity attributable to the amikacin was noted in the report. This is in contrast to the report by Benson from Chicago who reported the treatment of 20 patients with disseminated MAC infection with amikacin 15 mg/kg/day plus clofazamine, rifampin, ethambutol, and ciprofloxacin.[131] Nineteen of 20 patients had a favorable clinical and microbiological response. Two patients had recurrence of mycobacteremia with discontinuation of the amikacin, which was continued for a mean of 45.3 days. Three patients developed "severe ototoxicity" after receiving amikacin for more than 60 days.

Despite these encouraging reports, no controlled trials have been published, nor is there definite evidence of a decrease in mortality in treated patients. In most series, disseminated MAC has rarely been considered to be the cause of patients' death.[71,73,112] Horsburgh from the CDC presented life table analysis of data suggesting that AIDS patients with disseminated MAC have a shorter survival time (median, 7.4 months) compared to other AIDS patients with comparable degrees of immunosuppression (median, 13.3 months).[69] This was supported by a case-control study of HIV-seropositive patients with disseminated MAC matched for CD4 count, prior antiretroviral therapy, prior AIDS status, and year of diagnosis with HIV seropositive controls in which patients with untreated MAC infection had a significantly shorter survival (median, 4.1 months vs 11.1 months).[132] Additionally, this study showed that the survival of patients with disseminated MAC infection who received treatment with three or more antimycobacterial medications did not differ from that of the control patients. This is the first study to suggest that antimycobacterial therapy may prolong survival in AIDS patients with disseminated MAC infection and has implications for the design of future prospective controlled trials of antimycobacterial regimens in disseminated MAC infection.

There are several new agents that offer promise for more effective therapy of MAC infection. Liposomal preparations of aminoglycosides (both amikacin and gentamicin) have been shown to have improved bactericidal activity in the beige mouse model compared to free drug.[133,134] Liposomes tend to concentrate within macrophages in the reticuloendothelial system and should be particularly effective in the treatment of an intracellular pathogen such as MAC. In addition, liposomal preparations are less toxic and are cleared more slowly, potentially allowing for less frequent dosing as compared with free aminoglycosides.[134]

Several new macrolide compounds have significant in vitro activity against most MAC strains.[135] Azithromycin

A recent case-control study was the first to suggest that antimycobacterial therapy may prolong survival in AIDS patients with disseminated MAC infection.

It seems likely that combinations of more active drugs will be necessary to significantly alter the morbidity and mortality associated with disseminated MAC infection.

has been shown to be active in vitro and in the beige mouse model of MAC infection, decreasing mortality from 45% to 5% with oral administration over a 4-week period.[136] Azithromycin has very low serum concentrations but high tissue concentrations (and a long half-life) without significant toxicity.[136] Clarithromycin is another macrolide with in vitro activity against MAC, including activity within human macrophages where it was as active as rifabutin.[135,137] In pilot human studies, clarithromycin administration was associated with clearance of mycobacteremia in five of seven patients with HIV infection treated with clarithromycin alone, with two log reductions in colony-forming units in the other two patients.[138] Four patients receiving placebo had continuous bacteremia without any decrease in colony counts. It seems likely that combinations of more active drugs will be necessary to significantly alter the morbidity and mortality associated with disseminated MAC infection.

Given the success of Pneumocystis carinii prophylaxis, there has been interest in whether MAC infection could be prevented by treating patients who are only colonized.[66,129] Three patients with MAC isolated only from the respiratory tract were treated with isoniazid, ethambutol, rifabutin, and clofazamine and remained free of mycobacteremia for 2, 5, and 8 months.[129] Two remained alive after 12 and 21 months of therapy, whereas four concurrent patients who were not treated developed disseminated disease and died within 1 month of detection of dissemination. The numbers are quite small and the patients were not randomized, making any definite conclusions difficult. Another intriguing, but inconclusive, study was reported from New York in which 22 patients with AIDS on the basis of previous opportunistic infections who had received rifabutin 300–900 mg/day as an antiretroviral drug were retrospectively compared to 184 concurrent patients at another institution with regard to development of a diagnosis of disseminated MAC infection.[139] There was a trend toward prolonged MAC free survival in the treated group who received drug for more than 30 days. Currently controlled trials are in progress with both rifabutin and clofazamine as single agents for prevention of MAC infection.

Since it is impossible to distinguish MAC from *M tuberculosis* until the cultured organisms are identified, all HIV-seropositive patients with positive acid-fast organisms identified in clinical specimens should be treated with a regimen that is active against *M tuberculosis* until a definitive identification is available.[47] Once the organism is identified as *M avium* complex, the decision of whether to treat depends upon whether the patient is symptomatic,

Since symptoms tend to improve within 2–4 weeks in most patients who have responded clinically to treatment, it may be reasonable to offer the patient a trial of therapy with discontinuation if there is no improvement in clinical status after 4 weeks.

TABLE 5   Recommended Regimen for HIV-Seropositive Adults With Disseminated *M avium* Complex Infection

Drug	Dose
Rifampin	600 mg/day or 450 mg if <50 kg
Ethambutol	15–25 mg/kg/day
Clofazimine	100 mg/day
Ciprofloxacin	750 mg 2×/day
+/− Amikacin	7.5–15 mg/kg/day intravenously*

* adjusted for renal function

whether the patient is at the end stage of his or her HIV infection with multiple opportunistic infections present, and upon the patient's wishes regarding intensive therapies with intravenous agents and other potentially toxic drugs.[68] Since symptoms tend to improve within 2–4 weeks in most patients who have responded clinically to treatment, it may be reasonable to offer the patient a trial of therapy with discontinuation if there is no improvement in clinical status after 4 weeks.

Although one specific regimen of currently available drugs cannot be strongly recommended over others, a reasonable regimen including agents that are currently available is listed in Table 5. Monitoring for toxicity of the various drugs used in treating MAC is complicated by the presence of other opportunistic infections and malignancies and concomitant medications used to treat them.[65,66]

OTHER MYCOBACTERIAL INFECTIONS

The clinical experience with infection in AIDS patients caused by mycobacteria other than *M tuberculosis* and *M avium* complex is limited and consists mostly of case reports. Less than 4% of cases of disseminated nontuberculous mycobacterial infection in AIDS patients reported to the CDC from June 1981 through August 1987 were infected with organisms other than *M avium* complex.[69] However, since only disseminated disease with *M avium* complex or *M kansasii* were reportable as AIDS-defining opportunistic infections prior to the revision of the case definition in late 1987, infection with other mycobacteria were likely underreported.[11]

M kansasii was the most frequent species, other than *M avium* complex, causing disseminated disease in AIDS patients, representing 2.9% of all cases of disseminated nontuberculous mycobacterial infections reported to the CDC.[69] In a series of 36 patients from Miami with nontuberculous mycobacterial infection, 11 (30%) had infection

M kansasii was the most frequent species other than **M avium** *complex causing disseminated disease in AIDS patients, representing 2.9% of all cases of disseminated nontuberculous mycobacterial infections reported to the CDC.*

with *M kansasii*.[40] However, since the data from these patients are not presented separately from the cases of *M avium* complex infection, no conclusions can be made regarding the clinical presentation. Case reports of patients with disseminated disease have noted a clinical presentation similar to that of MAC infection, with the organism isolated from sputum, bronchial secretions, stool, duodenal tissue, lymph nodes, bone marrow, pleural fluid, and blood cultures.[22,140–142] Although *M kansasii* is usually sensitive to rifampin, ethambutol, and streptomycin in vitro, the results of treatment with these agents plus isoniazid (to which it is variably sensitive) have generally been discouraging in patients with AIDS.[22,140,141]

M gordonae is generally considered a nonpathogenic environmental mycobacterial species. However, 11 cases of disseminated disease with *M gordonae* in AIDS patients were included in the CDC report of disseminated nontuberculous mycobacterial infections in AIDS.[69] A case report described a patient with fever and weakness who grew *M gordonae* from sputum and a bone marrow biopsy specimen and died approximately 9 months later, despite therapy with multiple antimycobacterial drugs.[143]

M xenopi is also an uncommon cause of disease in immunocompetent patients and has been isolated from tap water and from hot-water generators in hospitals from which nosocomial disease may occur.[144] Disseminated disease has been described in patients with AIDS, including isolation of the organism from sputum, liver biopsy, stool, blood, bone marrow biopsy specimens, and bronchial washings.[144,145]

M fortuitum and *M chelonei* are rapidly growing mycobacteria that are ubiquitous in the environment. Disseminated disease is seen in immunocompromised patients, including 10 reported patients with AIDS, 5 of whom had *M fortuitum* and 5 had *M chelonei*.[69] A case report of disseminated *M fortuitum* infection in an AIDS patient emphasized disseminated subcutaneous nodules with necrosis and ulceration, as well as marked lymphadenopathy.[146] This patient improved with therapy, including amikacin and cefoxitin, and lived for 18 months, but had exacerbations of systemic symptoms thought secondary to *M fortuitum*, requiring recurrent hospitalization. Neither *M fortuitum* nor *M chelonei* is susceptible to usual antituberculous agents, and both are best managed on the basis of antimicrobial susceptibility testing, including drugs such as amikacin, cefoxitin, erythromycin, doxycycline, ciprofloxacin, and imipenam.[147]

M haemophilum is an acid-fast bacillus that requires hemin or another source of iron for growth and grows optimally at 32° C.[148] It has been rarely isolated as a cause of human infection, but has now been reported as a cause of disease in four AIDS patients.[148–150] M haemophilum has been associated with tenosynovitis, violaceous subcutaneous nodules, and cutaneous ulcerations in AIDS patients and has been cultured from aspirates of these involved areas as well as from blood, lymph nodes, and vitreous material.[148–150] The organism appears to be susceptible to rifampin in vitro, but is generally resistant to isoniazid and ethambutol.[150] Results of therapy in AIDS patients have been disappointing, with persistence of positive cultures and clinical abnormalities despite multidrug regimens.[148,149] When acid-fast organisms are seen on aspirates or biopsy of skin or subcutaneous lesions in patients with AIDS, appropriate media should be inoculated for the recovery of M haemophilum.

M bovis has been described as a cause of disseminated infection in patients with AIDS after vaccination with bacille Calmet-Guérine (BCG).[151,152] Two case reports of patients with HIV infection who developed active disease with M bovis after being given BCG 30 years previously, supports the recommendation that BCG not be used in the United States and other developed countries.[153,154]

Other nontuberculous mycobacteria have been isolated rarely from patients with AIDS, including some reports of mixed infection with two organisms.[155] Recently, there was a report of an as-yet-unidentified mycobacterium causing fatal infection in a patient with AIDS.[156] It seems likely that given the extreme immunosuppression of patients with end-stage HIV infection, any mycobacterial species could cause disease. Thus, isolation of any nontuberculous mycobacteria should prompt the clinician to evaluate the patient further for evidence of disease before dismissing the organism as a colonizer.

M haemophilum *has been associated with tenosynovitis, violaceous subcutaneous nodules, and cutaneous ulcerations in AIDS patients.*

References

1. Centers for Disease Control: Update: tuberculosis elimination—United States. MMWR 39:153, 1990

2. Centers for Disease Control: Tuberculosis, final data—United States, 1986. MMWR 36:817, 1988

3. Centers for Disease Control: Tuberculosis—United States, 1985—and the possible impact of human T-lymphotropic virus type III/lymphadenopathy-associated virus infection. MMWR 35:74, 1986

4. Centers for Disease Control: Tuberculosis and acquired immunodeficiency syndrome—Florida. MMWR 35:587, 1986

5. Centers for Disease Control: Tuberculosis and acquired immunodeficiency syndrome—New York City. MMWR 36:785, 1987

6. Sunderham G, McDonald RJ, Maniatis T et al: Tuberculosis as a manifestation of the acquired immunodeficiency syndrome (AIDS). JAMA 256:362, 1986

7. Pitchenik AE, Fischl MA, Dickinson GM et al: Opportunistic infections and Kaposi's sarcoma among Haitians: evidence of a new acquired immunodeficiency state. Ann Intern Med 98:277, 1983

8. Pitchenik AE, Cole C, Russell BW et al: Tuberculosis, atypical mycobacteriosis, and the acquired immunodeficiency syndrome among Haitian and non-Haitian patients in south Florida. Ann Intern Med 101:641, 1984

9. Handwerger S, Mildvan D, Senie R, McKinley FW: Tuberculosis and the acquired immunodeficiency syndrome at a New York City Hospital: 1978–1985. Chest 91:176, 1987

10. Louie E, Rice LB, Holzman RS: Tuberculosis in non-Haitian patients with acquired immunodeficiency syndrome. Chest 90:542, 1986

11. Centers for Disease Control: Revision of the CDC surveillance case definition for acquired immunodeficiency syndrome. MMWR 36(Suppl 1):3S, 1987

12. Braun MM, Byers RH, Heyward WL et al: Acquired immunodeficiency syndrome and extrapulmonary tuberculosis in the United States. Arch Intern Med 150:1913, 1990

13. Chaisson RE, Schecter GF, Theuer CP et al: Tuberculosis in patients with the acquired immunodeficiency syndrome: clinical features, response to therapy, and survival. Am Rev Respir Dis 136:570, 1987

14. Torres RA, Sridhar M, Altholz J, Brickner PW: Human immunodeficiency virus infection among homeless men in a New York City shelter: association with *Mycobacterium tuberculosis* infection. Arch Intern Med 150:2030, 1990

15. Pitchenik AE, Burr J, Suarez M et al: Human T-cell lymphotrophic virus-III (HTLV-III) seropositivity and related disease among 71 consecutive patients in whom tuberculosis was diagnosed. Am Rev Respir Dis 135:875, 1987

16. Theuer CP, Hopewell PC, Elias D et al: Human immunodeficiency virus infection in tuberculosis patients. J Infect Dis 162:8, 1990

17. Barber TW, Craven DE, McCabe WR: Bacteremia due to mycobacterium tuberculosis in patients with human immunodeficiency virus infection: a report of 9 cases and a review of the literature. Medicine 69:375, 1990

18. Selwyn PA, Hartel D, Lewis VA et al: A prospective study of the risk of tuberculosis among intravenous drug users with human immunodeficiency virus infection. N Engl J Med 320:545, 1989

19. Harries AD: Tuberculosis and human immunodeficiency virus infection in developing countries. Lancet 335:387, 1990

20. Elliott AM, Luo N, Tembo G et al: Impact of HIV on tuberculosis in Zambia: a cross sectional study. Br Med J 301:412, 1990

21. Pitchenik AE: Tuberculosis control and the AIDS epidemic in developing countries. Ann Intern Med 113:89, 1990

22. Helbert M, Robinson D, Buchanan D et al: Mycobacterial infection in patients infected with the human immunodeficiency virus. Thorax 45:45, 1990

23. Bouza E, Martin-Scapa C, Bernaldo de Quiros JCL et al: High prevalence of tuberculosis in AIDS patients in Spain. Eur J Clin Microbiol Infect Dis 7:785, 1988

24. Seligmann M, Pinching AJ, Rosen FS et al: Immunology of human immunodeficiency virus infection and the acquired immunodeficiency syndrome. Ann Intern Med 107:234, 1987

25. Gartner S, Markovits P, Markovitz DM et al: The role of mononuclear phagocytes in HTLV-III/LAV infection. Science 233:215, 1986

26. Des Prez RM, Heim CR: Mycobacterium tuberculosis. p. 1877. In Mandell GL, Douglas RG, Bennett JE (eds): Principles and practice of infectious diseases. 3rd ed. Churchill Livingstone, New York, 1990

27. Chaisson RE, Slutkin G: Tuberculosis and human immunodeficiency virus infection. J Infect Dis 159:96, 1989

28. Kramer FK, Modilevsky T, Waliany AR et al: Delayed diagnosis of tuberculosis in patients with human immunodeficiency virus infection. Am J Med 89:451, 1990

29. Modilevsky T, Sattler FR, Barnes PF: Mycobacterial disease in patients with human immunodeficiency virus infection. Arch Intern Med 149:2201, 1989

30. Ezratty A, Gumaste V, Rose E et al: Pancreatic tuberculosis: a frequently fatal but potentially curable disease. J Clin Gastroenterol 12:74, 1990

31. Goodman P, Pinero SS, Rance RM et al: Mycobacterial esophagitis in AIDS. Gastrointest Radiol 14:103, 1989

32. Blodi BA, Johnson MW, McLeish MW, Gass JDM: Presumed choroidal tuberculosis in a human immunodeficiency virus infected host. Am J Opthalmol 108:605, 1989

33. Doll DC, Yarbro JW: Mycobacterial spinal cord abscess with an ascending polyneuropathy. Ann Intern Med 106:333, 1987

34. Mallolas J, Gatell JM, Rovira M et al: Vertebral arch tuberculosis in two human immunodeficiency virus-seropositive heroin addicts. Arch Intern Med 148:1125, 1988

35. Lombardo PC, Weitzman I: Isolation of *Mycobacterium tuberculosis* and *M avium* complex from the same skin lesions in AIDS. N Engl J Med 323:916, 1990

36. Levy RM, Bredesen DE, Rosenblum ML: Opportunistic central nervous system pathology in patients with AIDS. Ann Neurol 23(Suppl):S7, 1988

37. Bishburg E, Sunderam G, Reichman LB, Kapila R: Central nervous system tuberculosis with the acquired immunodeficiency syndrome and its related complex. Ann Intern Med 105:210, 1986

38. Khan MA, Kovat DM, Bachus B et al: Clinical and roentgenographic spectrum of pulmonary tuberculosis in the adult. Am J Med 62:31, 1977

39. Pitchenik AE, Rubinson HA: The radiographic appearance of tuberculosis in patients with the acquired immune deficiency syndrome (AIDS) and Pre-AIDS. Am Rev Respir Dis 131:393, 1985

40. Fournier AM, Dickinson GM, Erdfrocht IR et al: Tuberculosis and nontuberculous mycobacteriosis in patients with AIDS. Chest 93:772, 1988

41. Centers for Disease Control: Diagnosis and management of mycobacterial infection and disease in persons with human immunodeficiency virus infection. Ann Intern Med 106:254, 1987

42. Daniel TM: Antibody and antigen detection for the immunodiagnosis of tuberculosis: why not? what more is needed? where do we stand today? J Infect Dis 158:678, 1988

43. Good RC: Serologic methods for diagnosing tuberculosis. Ann Intern Med 110:97, 1989

44. Murray JF, Mills J: Pulmonary infectious complications of human immunodeficiency virus infection. Am Rev Respir Dis 141:1356, 1990

45. Klein NC, Duncanson FP, Lenox TH et al: Use of mycobacterial smears in the diagnosis of pulmonary tuberculosis in AIDS/ARC patients. Chest 95:1190, 1989

46. Snider DE, Hopewell PC, Mills J, Reichman LB: Mycobacterioses and the acquired immunodeficiency syndrome. Am Rev Respir Dis 136:492, 1987

47. Prego V, Glatt AE, Roy V et al: Comparative yield of blood culture for fungi and mycobacteria, liver biopsy, and bone marrow biopsy in the diagnosis of fever of undetermined origin in human immunodeficiency virus-infected patients. Arch Intern Med 150:333, 1990

48. Hewlett D, Duncanson FP, Jagadha V et al: Lymphadenopathy in an inner-city population consisting principally of intravenous drug abusers with suspected acquired immunodeficiency syndrome. Am Rev Respir Dis 137:1275, 1988

49. Saltzman BR, Motyl MR, Friedland GH et al: *Mycobacterium tuberculosis* bacteremia in the acquired immunodeficiency syndrome. JAMA 256:390, 1986

50. Shafer RW, Goldberg R, Sierra M, Glatt AE: Frequency of *Mycobacterium tuberculosis* bacteremia in patients with tuberculosis in an area endemic for AIDS. Am Rev Respir Dis 140:1611, 1989

51. Witebsky FG, Keiser JF, Conville PS et al: Comparison of BACTEC 13A medium and DuPont isolator detection of mycobacteremia. J Clin Microbiol 26:1501, 1988

52. Colombrita D, Ravizzola G, Pinsi G et al: Rapid detection and identification of mycobacteria from blood of patients with acquired immune deficiency syndrome. J Med Microbiol 32:271, 1990

53. Iseman MD: Is standard chemotherapy adequate in tuberculosis patients infected with the HIV? Am Rev Respir Dis 136:1326, 1987

54. Small PM, Schecter GF, Goodman PC et al: Treatment of tuberculosis in patients with advanced human immunodeficiency virus infection. N Engl J Med 324:289, 1991

55. Centers for Disease Control: Screening for tuberculosis and tuberculous infection in high-risk populations, and the use of preventive therapy for tuberculous infection in the United States: recommendations of the Advisory Committee for Elimination of Tuberculosis. MMWR 39 (No RR-8): 1, 1990

56. Wadhawan D, Hira S, Mwansa N et al: Isoniazid prophylaxis among patients with HIV-I infection (abstract Th.B.510). In Abstracts from the VIth International Conference on AIDS. San Francisco, CA, 1990

57. Quinn TC: Interactions of the human immunodeficiency virus and tuberculosis and the implications for BCG vaccination. Rev Infect Dis 11 (Suppl):S379, 1989

58. Di Perri G, Cruciani M, Danzi MC et al: Nosocomial epidemic of active tuberculosis among HIV-infected patients. Lancet 2:1502, 1989

59. Centers for Disease Control: *Mycobacterium tuberculosis* transmission in a health clinic—Florida, 1988. MMWR 38:256, 1989

60. Centers for Disease Control: Nosocomial transmission of multidrug-resistant tuberculosis to health-care workers and HIV-infected patients in an urban hospital—Florida. MMWR 39:718, 1990

61. Wolinsky E: Nontuberculous mycobacteria and associated diseases. Am Rev Respir Dis 119:107, 1979

62. Horsburgh CR, Mason UG, Farhi DC, Iseman MD: Disseminated infection with *Mycobacterium avium-intracellulare*: a report of 13 cases and a review of the literature. Medicine 64:36, 1985

63. Greene JB, Sidhu GS, Lewin S et al: *Mycobacterium avium-intracellulare*: a cause of disseminated life threatening infection in homosexuals and drug abusers. Ann Intern Med 97:539, 1982

64. Zakowski P, Fligiel S, Berlin GW, Johnson Bl: Disseminated *Mycobacterium avium-intracellulare* infection in homosexual men dying of acquired immunodeficiency. JAMA 248:2980, 1982

65. Armstrong D, Gold JWM, Dryjanski J et al: Treatment of infections in patients with the acquired immunodeficiency syndrome. Ann Intern Med 103:738, 1985

66. Kaplan LD, Wofsy CB, Volberding PA: Treatment of patients with acquired immunodeficiency syndrome and associated manifestations. JAMA 257:1367, 1987

67. Glatt AE, Chirgwin K, Landesman SH: Treatment of infections associated with human immunodeficiency virus. N Engl J Med 318:1439, 1988

68. Young LS: *Mycobacterium avium* complex infection. J Infect Dis 157:863, 1988

69. Horsburgh CR, Selik RM: The epidemiology of disseminated nontuberculous mycobacterial infection in the acquired immunodeficiency syndrome (AIDS). Am Rev Respir Dis 139:4, 1989

70. Murray JF, Felton CP, Garay SM et al: Pulmonary complications of the acquired immunodeficiency syndrome: report of a National Heart, Lung, and Blood Institute workshop. N Engl J Med 310:1682, 1984

71. Hawkins CC, Gold JWM, Whimbey E et al: *Mycobacterium avium* complex infections in patients with the acquired immunodeficiency syndrome. Ann Intern Med 105:184, 1986

72. Macher AM, Kovacs JA, Gill V et al: Bacteremia due to *Mycobacterium avium-intracellulare* in the acquired immunodeficiency syndrome. Ann Intern Med 99:782, 1983

73. Hoy J, Mijch A, Sandland M et al: Quadruple-drug therapy for *Mycobacterium avium-intracellulare* bacteremia in AIDS patients. J Infect Dis 161:801, 1990

74. Young LS, Inderlied CB, Berlin OG, Gottlieb MS: Mycobacterial infections in AIDS patients, with an emphasis on the *Mycobacterium avium* complex. Rev Infect Dis 8:1024, 1986

75. Masur H. Tuazon C, Gill V et al: Effect of combined clofazemine and ansamycin therapy on *Mycobacterium avium-Mycobacterium intracellulare* bacteremia in patients with AIDS. J Infect Dis 155:127, 1987

76. Havlik JA, Horsburg CR, Metchock B et al: Clinical risk factors for disseminated *Mycobacterium avium* complex infection (DMAC) in persons with HIV infection (abstract Th. B. 515). In Abstracts from the VIth International Conference on AIDS. San Francisco, CA, 1990

77. Schurmann D, Ruf B, Mauch H, Pohle HD: Mycobacteremia in AIDS patients: results emphasizing the importance of routine blood culture (Abstract Th.B.513). In Abstracts from the VIth International Conference on AIDS. San Francisco, CA, 1990

78. Okello DO, Sewankambo N, Goodgame R et al: Absence of bacteremia with *Mycobacterium avium-intracellulare* in Ugandan patients with AIDS. J Infect Dis 162:208, 1990

79. O'Brien RJ: The epidemiology of nontuberculous mycobacterial disease. Clin Chest Med 10:407, 1989

80. Yakrus MA, Good RC: Geographic distribution, frequency, and specimen source of *Mycobacterium avium* complex serotypes isolated from patients with acquired immunodeficiency syndrome. J Clin Microbiol 28:926, 1990

81. Guthertz LS, Damsker B, Bottone EJ et al: *Mycobacterium avium* and *Mycobacterium intracellulare* infections in patients with and without AIDS. J Infect Dis 160:1037, 1989

82. Damsker B, Bottone EJ: *Mycobacterium avium-intracellulare* from the intestinal tracts of patients with the acquired immunodeficiency syndrome: concepts regarding acquisition and pathogenesis. J Infect Dis 151:179, 1985

83. Meissner PS, Falkinham Jo: Plasmid DNA profiles as epidemiological markers for clinical and environmental isolates of *Mycobacterium avium, Mycobacterium intracellulare,* and *Mycobacterium scrofulaceum.* J Infect Dis 153:325, 1986

84. Katz P, Yeager H, Whalen G et al: Natural killer cell-mediated lysis of *Mycobacterium-avium* complex-infected monocytes. J Clin Immunol 10:71, 1990

85. Crowle AJ, Cohn DL, Poche P: Defects in sera from acquired immunodeficiency syndrome (AIDS) patients and from non-AIDS patients with *Mycobacterium avium* infection which decrease macrophage resistance to *M. avium*. Infect Immun 57:1445, 1989

86. Wallace JM, Hannah JB: *Mycobacterium avium* complex infection in patients with acquired immunodeficiency syndrome: a clinicopathologic study. Chest 93:926, 1988

87. Connolly GM, Shanson D, Hawkins DA et al: Non-cryptosporidial diarrhoea in human immunodeficiency virus (HIV) infected patients. Gut 30:195, 1989

88. Roth RI, Owen RL, Keren DF, Volberding PA: Intestinal infection with *Mycobacterium avium* in acquired immune deficiency syndrome (AIDS): histological and clinical comparison with Whipple's disease. Dig Dis Sci 30:497, 1985

89. Gillin JS, Urmacher C, West R, Shike M: Disseminated *Mycobacterium avium-intracellulare* infection in acquired immunodeficiency syndrome mimicking Whipple's disease. Gastroenterology 85:1187, 1983

90. Schneebaum CW, Novick DM, Chabon AB et al: Terminal ileitis associated with *Mycobacterium avium-intracellulare* infection in a homosexual man with acquired immune deficiency syndrome. Gastroenterology 92:1127, 1987

91. Marinelli DL, Albelda SM, Williams TM et al: Nontuberculous mycobacterial infection in AIDS: clinical, pathologic, and radiographic features. Radiology 160:77, 1986

92. Tenholder MF, Moser RJ, Tellis CJ: Mycobacteria other than tuberculosis: pulmonary involvement in patients with acquired immunodeficiency syndrome. Arch Intern Med 148:953, 1988

93. Packer SJ, Cesario T, Williams JH: *Mycobacterium avium* complex infection presenting as endobronchial lesions in immunosuppressed patients. Ann Intern Med 109:389, 1988

94. Barbaro DJ, Orcutt VL, Coldiron BM: *Mycobacterium avium-Mycobacterium intracellulare* infection limited to the skin and lymph nodes in patients with AIDS. Rev Infect Dis 4:625, 1989

95. Snider WD, Simpson DM, Nielson S et al: Neurological complications of acquired immune deficiency syndrome: analysis of 50 patients. Ann Neurol 14:403, 1983

96. Cohen JI, Saragas SJ: Endophthalmitis due to *Mycobacterium avium* in a patient with AIDS. Ann Opthalmol 22:47, 1990

97. Woods GL, Goldsmith JC: Fatal pericarditis due to *Mycobacterium avium-intracellulare* in acquired immunodeficiency syndrome. Chest 95:1355, 1989

98. Kiehn TE, Edwards FF, Brannon P et al: Infections caused by *Mycobacterium avium* complex in immunocompromised patients: diagnosis by blood culture and fecal examination, antimicrobial susceptibility tests, and morphological and seroagglutination characteristics. J Clin Micro 21:168, 1985

99. Strand CL, Epstein C, Verzosa S et al: Evaluation of a new blood culture medium for mycobacteria. Am J Clin Path 91:316, 1989

100. Kiehn TE, Cammarata R: Comparative recoveries of *Mycobacterium avium-M intracellulare* from isolator lysis centrifugation and BACTEC 13A blood culture systems. J Clin Microbiol 26:760, 1988

101. Wong B, Edwards FF, Kiehn TE et al: Continuous high-grade *Mycobacterium avium-intracellulare* bacteremia in patients with the acquired immune deficiency syndrome. Am J Med 78:35, 1985

102. Eng RH, Bishburg E, Smith S, Mangia A: Diagnosis of *Mycobacterium* bacteremia in patients with acquired immunodeficiency syndrome by direct examination of blood films. J Clin Microbiol 27:768, 1989

103. Nussbaum JM, Dealist C, Lewis W, Heseltine PNR: Rapid diagnosis by buffy coat smear of

disseminated *Mycobacterium avium* complex infection in patients with acquired immunodeficiency syndrome. J Clin Microbiol 28:631, 1990

104. Barnes PF, Arevalo C: Blood culture positivity patterns in bacteremia due to *Mycobacterium avium-intracellulare*. South Med J 81:1059, 1988

105. Yagupsky P, Menegus MA: Cumulative positivity rate of multiple blood cultures for *Mycobacterium avium-intracellulare* and *Cryptococcus neoformans* in patients with the acquired immunodeficiency syndrome. Arch Pathol Lab Med 114:923, 1990

106. Poropatich CO, Labriola AM, Tuazon CU: Acid-fast smear and culture of respiratory secretions, bone marrow, and stools as predictors of disseminated *Mycobacterium avium* complex infection. J Clin Microbiol 25:929, 1987

107. Uribe-Botero G, Prichard JG, Kaplowitz HJ: Bone marrow in HIV infection: a comparison of fluorescent staining and cultures in the detection of mycobacteria. Am J Clin Pathol 91:313, 1989

108. Cohen RJ, Samoszuk MK, Busch D et al: Occult infections with *M intracellulare* in bone-marrow biopsy specimens from patients with AIDS. N Engl J Med 308:1475, 1983

109. Schneiderman DJ, Arenson DM, Cello JP et al: Hepatic disease in patients with the acquired immune deficiency syndrome (AIDS). Hepatology 7:925, 1987

110. Stacey AR: Isolation of *Mycobacterium avium-intracellulare-scrofulaceum* complex from faeces of patients with AIDS. Br Med J 293:1194, 1986

111. Stover DE, White DA, Romano PA, Gellene RA: Diagnosis of pulmonary disease in acquired immunodeficiency syndrome (AIDS): role of bronchoscopy and bronchoalveolar lavage. Am Rev Respir Dis 130:659, 1984

112. Klatt EC, Jensen DF, Meyer PR: Pathology of *Mycobacterium avium-intracellulare* infection in acquired immunodeficiency syndrome. Hum Pathol 18:709, 1987

113. Jannotta FS, Sidawy MK: The recognition of mycobacterial infections by intraoperative cytology in patients with acquired immunodeficiency syndrome. Arch Pathol Lab Med 113:1120, 1989

114. Stanley MW, Horwitz CA, Burton LG, Weisser JA: Negative images of bacilli and mycobacterial infection: a study of fine-needle aspiration smears from lymph nodes in patients with AIDS. Diagn Cytopathol 6:118, 1990

115. Bach MC, Bagwell SP, Masur H: Utility of gallium imaging in the diagnosis of *Mycobacterium avium-intracellulare* infection in patients with the acquired immunodeficiency syndrome. Clin Nucl Med 11:175, 1986

116. Kramer EL, Sanger JJ, Garay SM et al: Gallium-67 scans of the chest in patients with acquired immunodeficiency syndrome. J Nucl Med 28:1107, 1987

117. Nyberg DA, Federle MP, Jeffrey RB et al: Abdominal CT findings of disseminated *Mycobacterium avium-intracellulare* in AIDS. AJR 145:297, 1985

118. Yajko DM, Nassos PS, Sanders CA, Hadley WK: Killing by antimycobacterial agents of AIDS-derived strains of *Mycobacterium avium* complex inside cells of the mouse macrophage cell line J774. Am Rev Respir Dis 140:1198, 1989

119. Heifets LB, Iseman MD: Choice of antimicrobial agents for *M. avium* disease based on quantitative tests of drug susceptibility. N Engl J Med 323:419, 1190

120. Inderlied CB, Young LS, Yamada JK: Determination of in vitro susceptibility of *Mycobacterium avium* complex isolates to antimycobacterial agents by various methods. Antimicrob Agents Chemother 31:1697, 1987

121. Heifets LB, Lindholm-Levy PJ, Flory MA: Bactericidal activity in vitro of various rifamycins against *Mycobacterium avium* and *Mycobacterium tuberculosis*. Am Rev Respir Dis 141:626, 1990

122. Hoffner SE, Kratz M, Olsson-Liljequist B et al: In-vitro synergistic activity between ethambutol and fluorinated quinolones against *Mycobacterium avium* complex. J Antimicrob Chemother 24:317, 1989

123. Rastogi N, Goh KS, David HL: Enhancement of drug susceptibility of *Mycobacterium avium* by inhibitors of cell envelope synthesis. Antimicrob Agents Chemother 34:759, 1990

124. Yajko DM, Kirihara J, Sanders C et al: Antimicrobial synergism against *Mycobacterium avium* complex strains isolated from patients with acquired immune deficiency syndrome. Antimicrob Agents Chemother 32:1392, 1988

125. Heifets S, Lindholm-Levy P: Comparison of bactericidal activities of streptomycin, amikacin, kanamycin, and capreomycin against *Mycobacterium avium* and *M. tuberculosis*. Antimicrob Agents Chemother 33:1298, 1989

126. Gangadharam PRJ, Perumal VK, Podapati NR et al: In vivo activity of amikacin alone or in combination with clofazamine or rifabutin or both against acute experimental *Mycobacterium avium* complex infections in beige mice. Antimicrob Agents Chemother 32:1400, 1988

127. Saito H, Sato K: Activity of rifabutin alone and in combination with clofazamine, kanamycin and ethambutol against *Mycobacterium intracellulare* infections in mice. Tubercle 70:201, 1989

128. Baron EJ, Young LS: Amikacin, ethambutol, and rifampin for treatment of disseminated *Mycobacterium avium-intracellulare* infections in patients with acquired immune deficiency syndrome. Diagn Microbiol Infect Dis 5:215, 1986

129. Agins BD, Berman DS, Spicehandler D et al: Effect of combined therapy with ansamycin, clofazamine, ethambutol, and isoniazid for *Mycobacterium avium* infection in patients with AIDS. J Infect Dis 159:784, 1989

130. Chiu J, Nussbaum J, Bozzette S et al: Treatment of disseminated *Mycobacterium avium* complex infection in AIDS with amikacin, ethambutol, rifampin, and ciprofloxacin. Ann Intern Med 113:358, 1990

131. Benson C, Pottage J, Kessler H: Treatment of AIDS-related disseminated *Mycobacterium avium* complex disease (DMAC) with a multiple drug regimen including amikacin (abstract Th. B. 517). In Abstracts from the VIth International Conference on AIDS. San Francisco, CA, 1990

132. Horsburg CR, Havlik JA, Thompson SE: Survival of AIDS patients with disseminated *Mycobacterium avium* complex infection (DMAC): a case-control study (abstract TH. B. 516). In Abstracts from the VIth International Conference on AIDS. San Francisco, CA, 1990

133. Cynamon MH, Swenson CE, Palmer GS, Ginsberg RS: Liposome-encapsulated-amikacin therapy of *Mycobacterium avium* complex infection in beige mice. Antimicrob Agents Chemother 33:1179, 1989

134. Bermudez LE, Yau-Young AO, Lin J-P et al: Treatment of disseminated *Mycobacterium avium* complex infection of beige mice with liposome-encapsulated aminoglycosides. J Infect Dis 161:1262, 1990

135. Naik S, Ruck R: In vitro activities of several new macrolide antibiotics against *Mycobacterium avium* complex. Antimicrob Agents Chemother 33:1614, 1989

136. Inderlied CB, Kolonoski PT, Wu M, Young LS: In vitro and in vivo activity of azithromycin (CP 62,993) against the *Mycobacterium avium* complex. J Infect Dis 159:994, 1989

137. Perronne C, Gikas A, Truffot-Pernot C et al: Activities of clarithromycin, sulfisoxazole, and rifabutin against, *Mycobacterium avium* complex multiplication within human macrophages. Antimicrob Agents Chemother 34:1508, 1990

138. Prokocimer P, Dellerson M, Craft C et al: Effect of clarithromycin (C) on blood cultures (BC) positive for *Mycobacterium avium* complex (MAC) in HIV + patients (abstract 634). In Abstracts of the 30th Interscience Conference on Antimicrobial Agents and Chemotherapy. Atlanta, GA, 1990

139. Siegal FP, Borenstein M, Gehan K et al: Rifabutin may delay the onset of *Mycobacterium avium* complex infection (MAC) in patients with AIDS (abstract Th.B. 518). In Abstracts from the VIth International Conference on AIDS. San Francisco, CA, 1990

140. Sherer R, Sable R, Sonnenberg M et al: Disseminated infection with *Mycobacterium kansasii* in the acquired immunodeficiency syndrome. Ann Intern Med 105:710, 1986

141. Hirasuna JD: Disseminated *Mycobacterium kansasii* infection in the acquired immunodeficiency syndrome (AIDS). Ann Intern Med 107:784, 1987

142. Truffot-Pernot C, Lecoeur HF, Maury L et al: Results of blood cultures for detection of mycobacteria in AIDS patients. Tubercle 70:187, 1989

143. Chan J, McKitrick JC, Klein RS: *Mycobacterium gordonae* in the acquired immunodeficiency syndrome. Ann Intern Med 101:400, 1984

144. Ausina V, Barrio J, Luquin M et al: *Mycobacterium xenopi* infections in the acquired immunodeficiency syndrome. Ann Intern Med 109:927, 1988

145. Tecson-Tumang FT, Bright JL: *Mycobacterium xenopi* and the acquired immunodeficiency syndrome. Ann Intern Med 100:461, 1984

146. Sack JB: Disseminated infection due to *Mycobacterium fortuitum* in a patient with AIDS. Rev Infect Dis 12:961, 1990

147. Wallace RJ, Swenson JA, Silcox VA et al: Treatment of nonpulmonary infections due to *Mycobacterium fortuitum* and *Mycobacterium chelonei* on the basis of in vitro susceptibilities. J Infect Dis 152:500, 1985

148. Males BM, West TE, Bartholomew WR: *Mycobacterium haemophilum* infection in a patient with acquired immune deficiency syndrome. J Clin Microbiol 25:136, 1987

149. Rogers Pl, Walker RE, Lane HC et al: Disseminated *Mycobacterium haemophilum* infection in two patients with the acquired immunodeficiency syndrome. Am J Med 84:640, 1988

150. Thibert L, Lebel F, Martineau B: Two cases of *Mycobacterium haemophilum* infection in Canada. J Clin Microbiol 28:621, 1990

151. Centers of Disease Control: Disseminated *Mycobacterium bovis* infection from BCG vaccination of a patient with acquired immunodeficiency syndrome. MMWR 34:227, 1985

152. Bouds P, Sobel A, Deforges L et al: Disseminated *Mycobacterium bovis* infection from BCG vaccination and HIV infection. JAMA 262:2386, 1989

153. Reynes J, Perez C, Lamaury I et al: Bacille Calmette-Guerin adenitis 30 years after immunization in a patient with AIDS. J Infect Dis 160:727, 1989

154. Armbruster C, Junker W, Vetter N, Jaksch G: Disseminated bacille Calmette-Guerin infection in an AIDS patient 30 years after BCG vaccination. J Infect Dis 162:1216, 1990

155. Levy-Frebault V, Pangon B, Bure A: *Mycobacterium simiae* and *Mycobacterium avium-M. intracellulare* mixed infection in acquired immune deficiency syndrome. J Clin Microbiol 25:154, 1987

156. Hirschel B, Chang HR, Mach N et al: Fatal infection with a novel, unidentified mycobacterium in a man with the acquired immunodeficiency syndrome. N Engl J Med 323:109, 1990

INDEX

Page numbers followed by the letter *f* refer to figures; those followed by *t* refer to tables.